Sleep – Physiology, Functions, Dreaming and Disorders Series

Sleep Apnea Syndrome from Clinical and Neurophysiological Aspects in the Stomatognathic System

SLEEP – PHYSIOLOGY, FUNCTIONS, DREAMING AND DISORDERS SERIES

Narcolepsy: Symptoms, Causes and Diagnosis
Guillermo Santos and Lautar Villalba (Editors)
2010. ISBN: 978-1-60876-645-1

Conditioned Arousal in Insomnia Patients
Aisha Cortoos, Elke De Valck, and Raymond Cluydts
2010. ISBN: 978-1-61668-421-1

Sleep Apnea Syndrome from Clinical and Neurophysiological Aspects in the Stomatognathic System
Kazuya Yoshida
2010. ISBN: 978-1-60876-985-8

SLEEP – PHYSIOLOGY, FUNCTIONS, DREAMING
AND DISORDERS SERIES

SLEEP APNEA SYNDROME FROM CLINICAL AND NEUROPHYSIOLOGICAL ASPECTS IN THE STOMATOGNATHIC SYSTEM

KAZUYA YOSHIDA

Nova Science Publishers, Inc.
New York

Copyright © 2010 by Nova Science Publishers, Inc.

All rights reserved. No part of this book may be reproduced, stored in a retrieval system or transmitted in any form or by any means: electronic, electrostatic, magnetic, tape, mechanical photocopying, recording or otherwise without the written permission of the Publisher.

For permission to use material from this book please contact us:
Telephone 631-231-7269; Fax 631-231-8175
Web Site: http://www.novapublishers.com

NOTICE TO THE READER
The Publisher has taken reasonable care in the preparation of this book, but makes no expressed or implied warranty of any kind and assumes no responsibility for any errors or omissions. No liability is assumed for incidental or consequential damages in connection with or arising out of information contained in this book. The Publisher shall not be liable for any special, consequential, or exemplary damages resulting, in whole or in part, from the readers' use of, or reliance upon, this material.

Independent verification should be sought for any data, advice or recommendations contained in this book. In addition, no responsibility is assumed by the publisher for any injury and/or damage to persons or property arising from any methods, products, instructions, ideas or otherwise contained in this publication.

This publication is designed to provide accurate and authoritative information with regard to the subject matter covered herein. It is sold with the clear understanding that the Publisher is not engaged in rendering legal or any other professional services. If legal or any other expert assistance is required, the services of a competent person should be sought. FROM A DECLARATION OF PARTICIPANTS JOINTLY ADOPTED BY A COMMITTEE OF THE AMERICAN BAR ASSOCIATION AND A COMMITTEE OF PUBLISHERS.

LIBRARY OF CONGRESS CATALOGING-IN-PUBLICATION DATA

Yoshida, Kazuya, 1960-
Sleep apnea syndrome in the stomatognathic system / Kazuya Yoshida.
  p. cm.
Includes index.
ISBN 978-1-60876-985-8 (softcover)
1. Sleep apnea syndromes. I. Title.
RC737.5.Y67 2009
616.2'09--dc22
                                                                2009050566

Published by Nova Science Publishers, Inc. ✤ *New York*

CONTENTS

Preface		vii
Chapter 1	Clinical Aspects of Sleep Apnea Syndrome	1
Chapter 2	Neurophysiological Aspect of Sleep Apnea Syndrome	51
Conclusion		91
References		93
Index		113

PREFACE

Obstructive sleep apnea is a disorder characterized by repetitive, complete or partial closure of the upper airway during sleep. Obstructive sleep apnea syndrome is related to different combinations of anatomical and functional aspects that produce the airway collapse in individual patients.

To compensate for the craniofacial abnormalities and treat sleep apnea syndrome, there are some dental or maxillofacial surgical modalities such as oral appliance, orthognathic surgery or distraction osteogenesis. Of these options, the oral appliance is an important treatment choice and may be the preferred initial treatment for mild to moderate obstructive sleep apnea syndrome or snoring. Its effects on respiratory function and sleep quality variables, and factors influencing these effects are discussed. Prevention of the syndrome has rarely been considered, but orthodontic treatment for children with micrognathia and even habitual sufficient chewing can lead to normal craniofacial growth and development and may be able to prevent airway obstruction from developing.

The neurophysiological effect of the stomatognathic system function on sleep apnea syndrome remains uncertain. Electromyograms (surface or intramuscular) have been used to study the jaw and upper airway muscles during sleep. Electroencephalograms (movement-related cortical potentials or contingent negative variation) were used to elucidate the role of the cerebral cortex in the control of movements and the cognitive process in preparation for a response directed to a purpose. Recent advances in functional brain-imaging techniques such as magnetoencephalography and near-infrared spectroscopy have enabled examination of brain activity during various tasks. These methods can provide important information on the neurophysiological basis of sleep breathing disorders. The stomatognathic system can affect sleep apnea syndrome both anatomically and functionally. Further studies from the standpoint of stomatognathic system will be necessary.

Chapter 1

CLINICAL ASPECTS OF SLEEP APNEA SYNDROME

1. SLEEP APNEA SYNDROME

a. Definition

Sleep apnea is defined as 30 or more apneic episodes (the cessation of airflow at the mouth and nose for more than 10 s) [1]. Typical subjective complaints of SAS are excessive daytime sleepiness, loud and irregular snoring, disturbed nighttime sleep, mental deterioration and depression. Collapse between the base of the tongue and adjacent posterior and lateral pharyngeal wall is the most prevalent site of airway closure [2]. The obstruction may occur also at the level of the soft palate if it is particularly long. These anatomical factors, combined with a functional loss of muscle tone in the upper airway during sleep, result in obstruction of the airway due to the negative pressure exerted by continued diaphragmatic effort. Periods of apnea frequently last 10 to 30 s, and some continue for more than 100 s. Without adequate ventilation, the blood carbon dioxide pressure eventually increases to a level that arouses the patient. The patient wakens briefly, inhales, and then returns to sleep, without consciously remembering the episode. This sleep pattern disturbance repeats itself throughout the night. As a result of the disturbed sleep, excessive daytime somnolence, cognitive dysfunction and memory loss occur. This has significant sequelae in the professional and social world. In addition, the patients with this condition are at increased risk of death from automobile accidents [3]. A definitive diagnosis of SAS is made by polysomnography. Indicators of the condition include obesity, particularly increased collar size and the above-mentioned symptoms. Sleep apnea is classified into three types; obstructive, central and mixed. Obstructive apnea is the most common type, and results from collapse or obstruction of the oropharyngeal region of the upper airway. Central apnea is characterized by the simultaneous cessation of both airflow and respiratory effort. During mixed apnea, a central respiratory pause is followed by an obstructed ventilatory effort. The SAS is a relatively common and potentially lethal disorder, with an estimated prevalence of approximately 4 % for the middle-aged adult population [4]. It is associated with an increased prevalence of cardiovascular complications, such as arterial hypertension [5], coronary artery disease [6], and nocturnal angina [7].

b. Craniofacial Morphology and SAS

Narrowing or obstruction of upper airway are affected by morpohological factors of the craniofacial structure such as abnormally narrow upper airways, long velum palatinum, tonsillar and adenoid hypertrophy, micrognathia and retrognathia, nasal insufficiency, fat infiltration of the oropharynx, open mandibular angle, hypertrophy and thickness of the tongue, and lowered hyoid bone [8]. Non-obese SAS patients, often observed in the Japanese population, tend to show skeletal abnormality. On the other hand, obese SAS patients have a tendency to abnormality of the soft tissue. Asians suffer from SAS more easily than Europeans and Americans due to characteristics of their craniofacial morphology, even if they are not so obese [9]. Therefore, it is important to research SAS treatment in Japan. The ratio of the maximum breadth to the maximum length of the skull, multiplied by 100 is called the cranial index and is used to evaluate the form of the skull in anatomy and anthropology. A dolichocephalic (long-headed) person has a cranial index of less than 75. A brachycephalic (short-headed) person has a cranial index between 80 and 85. When we look at the head from the upper part, the head is long antero-posteriorly if the cranial index is low in dolichocephalic people. The head is round if the index is high in brachycephalic people.

On cephalometric exams in normal patients, the tangent to the inferior border of the mandible usually passes inferior to the cranium. In cases with a steep mandibular angle, the tangent often passes into the cranium. The so-called "long face syndrome" is often associated with crossbite, tension nose, and a Class-II (mandibular retrognathic) occlusion. Any condition that causes nasal obstruction such as a deviated septum, hypertrophic turbinates or external nasal deformity could lead to this typical facial morphology. This syndrome is characterized by an increased vertical facial height in the lower third of the face, excessive dentoalveolar height, a high arched palate and a steep mandibular plane. Patients with long face syndrome tend to have problems breathing through their nose as their sinus cavities tend to be narrow, inhibiting airflow. Consequently, these patients tend to breathe through their mouth, a contributing factor for some people who snore or who suffer from sleep apnea. Orthodontic appliances can widen the face and mouth, which in turn widens the sinus cavities, allowing easier nasal breathing. Generally, the Japanese tend to be brachycephal with a long face compared with Caucasians (Figure 1). In a person with a short face who is dolichocephal, the skull is long antero-posteriorly and short superior-inferiorly. The pharyngeal space is thick and short, so obstructions occur [9]. On the other hand, in a person with long face who is brachycephal, the skull is short antero-posteriorly and long supero-inferiorly. The pharyngeal space is narrow and long, so a collapse can occur easily (Figure 1).

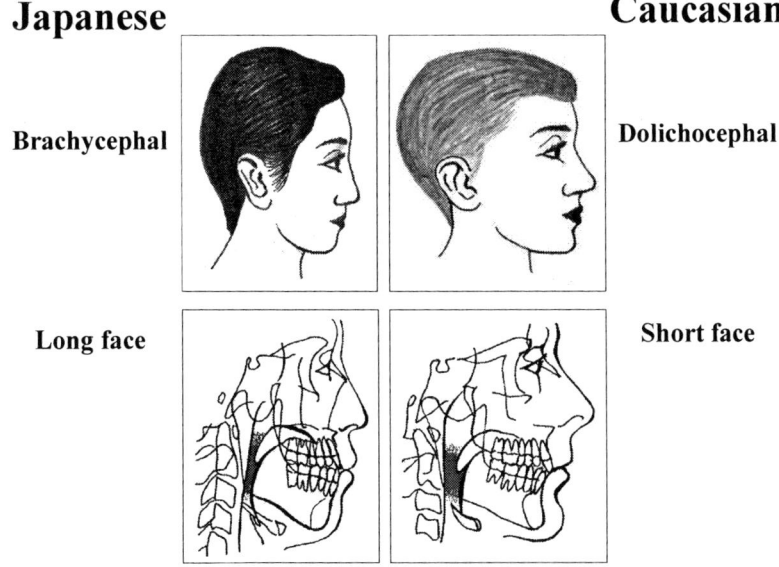

Figure 1. Difference in craniofacial morphology between Japanese and Caucasian. Generally the Japanese has a tendency to brachycephal and long face compared with Caucasians. In a person with a short face and dolichocephal morphology, the skull is long antero-posteriorly and short superior-inferiorly. The pharyngeal space is thick and short, and therefore obstruction hardly occurs. On the other hand, in a person with a long face and brachycephal, the skull is short antero-posteriorly and long supero-inferiorly. The pharyngeal space is narrow and long, and consequently a collapse can occur easily.

c. Chewing and SAS

Craniofacial growth and development are influenced by heredity and also environmental factors like chewing. The number of chewing times per meal of modern Japanese is thought to be about 600. It was estimated to be about 1,400 times with prewar Japanese food, and it is thought that chewing about 4,000 times was necessary in the Yayoi period (BC 1000-AD 300).

It is thought that chewing traditional Japanese food or hard food thoroughly promoted the development of craniofacial morphology such as the masticatory muscles and jawbone [9].

Maxillary alveolar length and width increased slightly (Figure 2), while mandibular alveolar length and width decreased gradually (Figure 3) [10]. Decreasing the number of chewing actions slows maturity of the craniofacial morphology, but tooth size does not change so there is no room for teeth to erupt and youths with impacted teeth have increased (Figure 4).

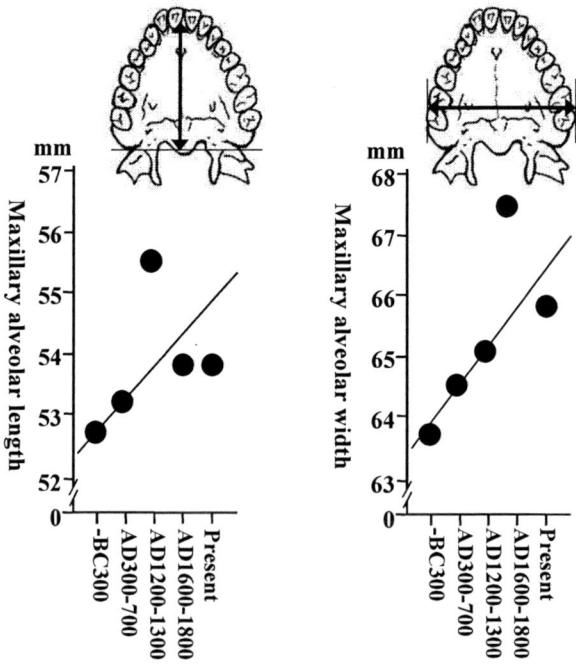

Figure 2. Changes in maxillar length and width in Japanese from BC 300 to the present. The maxillary length and width increased slightly.

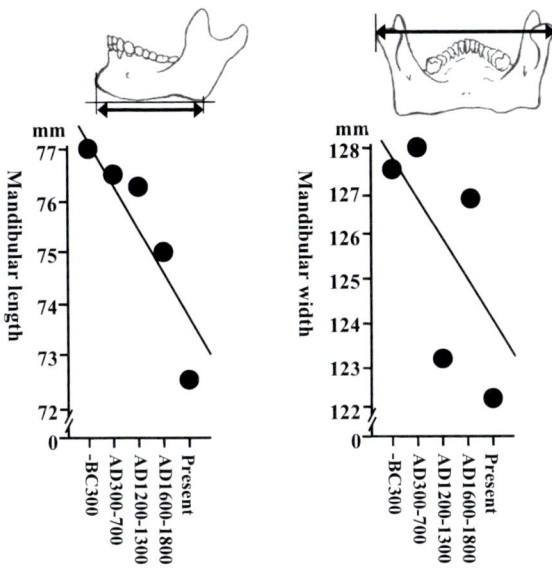

Figure 3. Changes in mandibular length and width. The mandibular length and width decreased gradually.

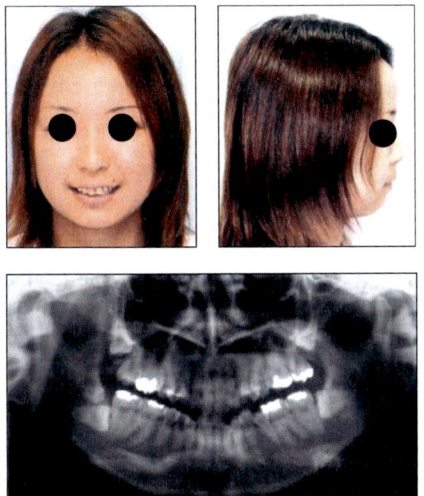

Figure 4. A nineteen-year old female with micrognathia. Despite her small maxilla and mandible the number and size of teeth do not decrease. Note the impacted fourth molar distal of the right lower impacted third molar. Due to the rapid decrease of number of chewing times, such youths are increasing.

There is a tendency towards such micrognathia or malocclusion in the onset of SAS after middle age, and an increase in SAS resulting from immature morphology in the future is expected. Fatty and soft foods such as fatty tuna have become popular. The quantity of saliva secretion increases if we chew food sufficiently, and the satiety center is stimulated; it is thought that this restrains overeating and therefore obesity. Immaturity of the craniofacial structure due to a decrease in the number of chewing actions and obesity as a result of eating high calorie Western foods will lead to more SAS in the future, and this is a concern. No attention has been paid to the prevention of SAS at all, but habitual chewing from childhood promotes normal growth of craniofacial morphology, restrains overeating and obesity and may prevent SAS.

2. TREATMENT

The treatment for SAS includes conservative methods, such as weight loss therapy [11], positional therapy [12], oral appliance therapy [13-22], use of continuous positive airway pressure (CPAP) [23-25], surgical methods such as uvulopalatopharyngoplasty [26], maxillomandibular advancement surgery [27] and tracheostomy [28]. Weight loss and positional therapies have been largely unsatisfactory. A variety of oral appliances have been effectively used for the treatment of sleep apnea syndrome [29-32]. All are constructed with the goal of advancing the position of the mandible and tongue in order to enlarge the airway or reduce its collapsibility (Figures 5, 6). The American Sleep Disorders Association has issued guidelines which state that oral appliance therapy is indicated for snoring, for mild obstructive sleep apnea, and for moderate to severe sleep apnea if CPAP is not accepted or if surgery is not appropriate [33]. CPAP is a very effective treatment. However, problems associated with CPAP use leading to non-compliance include nasal congestion, discomfort secondary to pressure sensation and air-leak, and mask intolerance. Its long-term use is 50 to 80 %, and patients with slight symptoms are more likely to discontinue treatment [34, 35]. Crossover studies comparing the efficacy of CPAP and oral appliance reported that the oral appliances were effective for obstructive sleep apnea, especially for mild-moderate cases, and associated with fewer side effects and greater patient satisfaction than CPAP [34, 35]. Conventional surgical management for pediatric obstructive sleep apnea is adenotonsillectomy. Patients with severe sleep apnea may require uvulopalatopharyngoplasty to relieve their obstruction. Failure of uvulopalatopharyngoplasty to relieve the obstruction may require tracheostomy or mandibular advancement.

Clinical Aspects of Sleep Apnea Syndrome

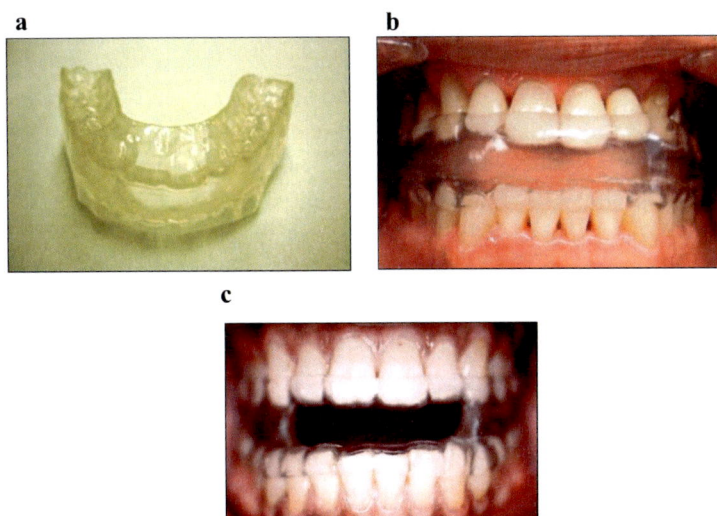

Figure 5. Oral appliances for the treatment of SAS or snoring. Rigid type mandibular repositioning appliance without anterior opening (a,b) and with it (c).

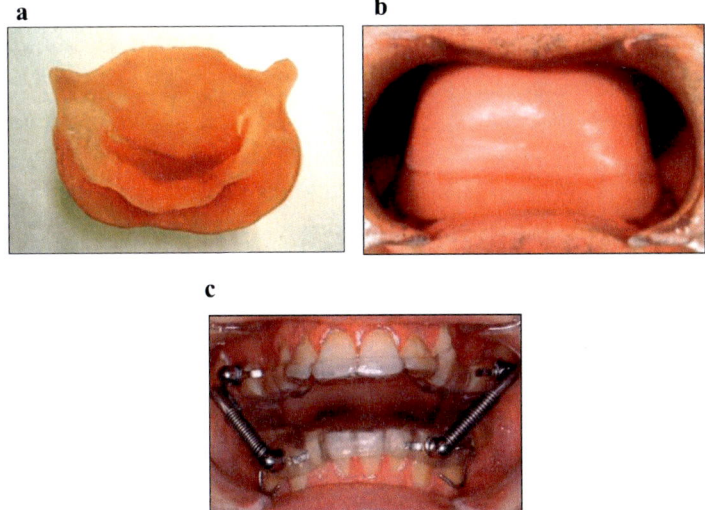

Figure 6. Tongue retaining device (a,b), and adjustable appliance with Herbst attachments (c) for the treatment of SAS or snoring. The Herbst appliance (c) permits jaw protrusive opening, and some limited side-to-side movement, but no retrusive movement. To use the tongue retaining device (a,b) the patient advances the tongue into the anterior bulb (b) while squeezing the bulb to create negative suction.

These surgical treatments involve possible complications such as postoperative stenosis, pain and infection. Moreover, life-threatening complications such as airway obstruction and serious arrhythmias are occasionally observed peri- and postoperatively. The efficacies of the surgical therapies range from 30 to 50 % [36, 37]. Surgical treatment should be restricted to those patients who have severe effects of the syndrome and whose sleep apnea is resistant to conservative treatment because of complications and relatively low success rates.

a. Oral Appliance Therapy

Patients with an apnea-hypopnea index (AHI) of more than 30 demonstrate significant neuropsychological morbidity which is improved by CPAP therapy [24, 25]. However the optimal management mode and treatment benefits for mild to moderate SAS remain inconclusive. Oral appliances can be divided into two main groups: mandibular advancement appliances and tongue retaining device. The first category is by far the most common type of appliance in use today. The protrusion distance of these devices can be fixed or variable. The second group, tongue retaining device, is applied seldom; mainly if there are dental reasons, i.e. the patient is edentulous, precluding the construction of a mandibular advancement appliance. Another category is the palatal lifting device. This contacts the soft palate directly, but is no longer in use today. Since Meier-Ewert et al. [13] (1984) first described treatment of sleep apnea by a mandibular protracting device (Esmarch device), the device and a modified Esmarch appliance [22, 38] have been effectively used for the treatment of sleep apnea [19, 22, 39]. The device postures the mandible at an elevated vertical and protrusive position. The mandibular position may be adjusted, if necessary, after initial construction by separating the maxillary and mandibular splints.

Of a variety of mandibular advancing devices, rigid appliances restrict mandibular movements, while the Herbst appliance permits jaw protrusive opening, and some limited side-to-side movement, but no retrusive movement (Figure 6c). The Herbst appliance consists of separate maxillary and mandibular appliances, intra-arch elastics and lateral tube and rod attachments (Herbst attachment). This appliance has been used in orthodontics and also for sleep apnea treatment. The elastics, tubes and attachments are attached to both buccal sides of the maxillary and mandibular appliances. This can result in discomfort of the buccal mucosa. More recently, an elastic retracted oral appliance was reported [40]. The appliance allows free mandibular movement and can be used to treat sleep apnea in mentally impaired patients and patients with neuromuscular disabilities. Klearway facilitates very slow and gradual movement of the mandible by permitting the patient to adjust the appliance according to his or her own comfort level with the guidance of the attending dentist [41]. The snore guard is a boil-and-bite appliance that is easy to fit and adjust directly on the patient and appears to be well tolerated. The appliance is used only for the treatment of snoring. The tongue retaining device has an anterior bulb which, by means of negative pressure, holds the tongue forward during sleep [42] (Figure 6a, b). It is an alternative to a mandibular repositioner in patients with compromised dentition or who are edentulous.

Oral appliance therapy provides an important treatment choice and may be the preferred initial treatment. However, most studies have dealt with limited sleep parameters in a small size of patients. In addition some appliances require special orthodontic attachment and must be fabricated in orthodontic laboratories. It seems meaningful to introduce a simplified appliance which can be made easily in every dental laboratory, and to evaluate the respiratory function and sleep quality variables in a larger size of patients [22].

The appliance, which the author has used most frequently, is fabricated individually for each patient as follows [22]. Impressions of maxillary and mandibular dental arches are taken with alginate impression material. The maximal protrusive distance of movement measured from the position of maximum intercuspation without any discomfort is checked and measured. The degree of mandibular advancement was 60 to 80 % of each patient's maximum protrusive distance (Figures 7, 8). Mandibular advancement ranged between 3.0 and 10.0 mm, and mandibular opening (bite raising) between 6.0 and 12 mm. Some studies showed that greater amounts of mandibular protrusion are related to greater reductions in respiratory events [20, 43], although the effects of the amount of vertical opening on effect and complications remain uncertain. We use a simple method, the "quasi-snoring sound test", to determine the optimal mandibular position. The patient is requested to perform quasi-snoring by inspirating air through nose on a horizontally-reclined dental chair (Figure 9). We gradually protrude the patient's mandible by hand. The position where the patient's snoring sound disappears should be the most preferable protrusion distance. Occasionally the sound does not disappear at the maximal protrusion. If so, an oral appliance would not improve sleep-disordered breathing. As an anatomical problem in the nasopharynx might be present, the patient is referred to an otorynolaryngologist. An interocclusal record is taken using silicone paste (Lab Silicone, Shofu, Kyoto, Japan) in the bilateral premolar and molar area (Figure 7). At that time the interocclusal relationship at a protrusive and elevated vertical position is checked in the incisal area.

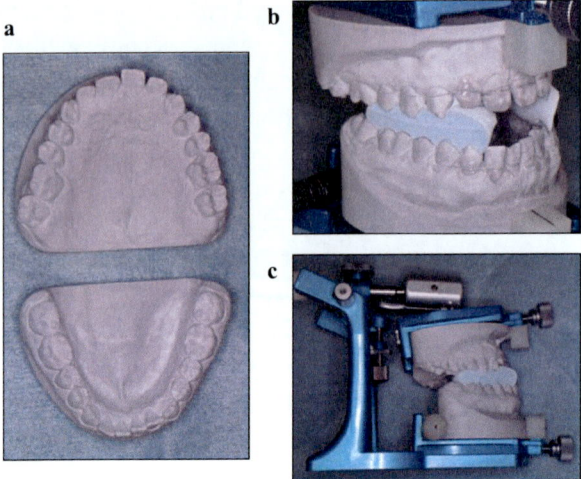

Figure 7. Plaster models of maxillary and mandibular dental arches (a). The degree of mandibular advancement was 60 to 80 % of each patient's maximum protrusive distance (b). The master casts and splints were mounted in the articulator using the interocclusal record (c).

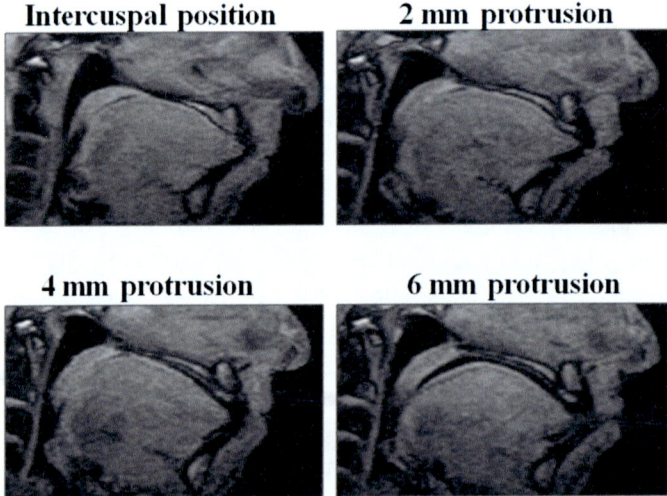

Figure 8. Change in caliber of upper airway associated mandibular advancement measured by sagittal slice of MRI. The advancement for an effective oral appliance must be 4-5mm based on the space between soft palate or tongue base and posterior pharyngeal wall.

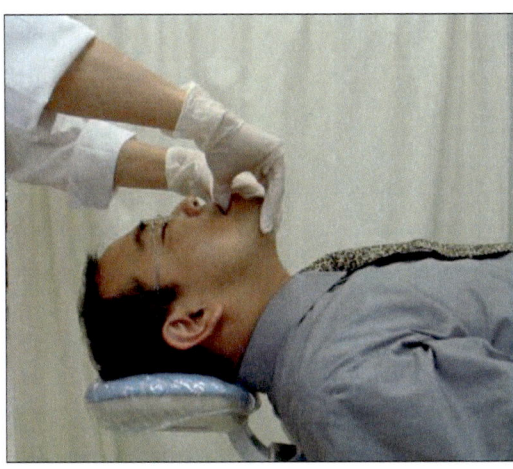

Figure 9. Quasi-snoring sound test. The patient is requested to perform quasi-snoring by inspirating air through their nose on a horizontally reclined dental chair. We gradually protrude the patient's mandible by hand. The position where patient's snoring sound disappears should be the most preferable protrusion distance.

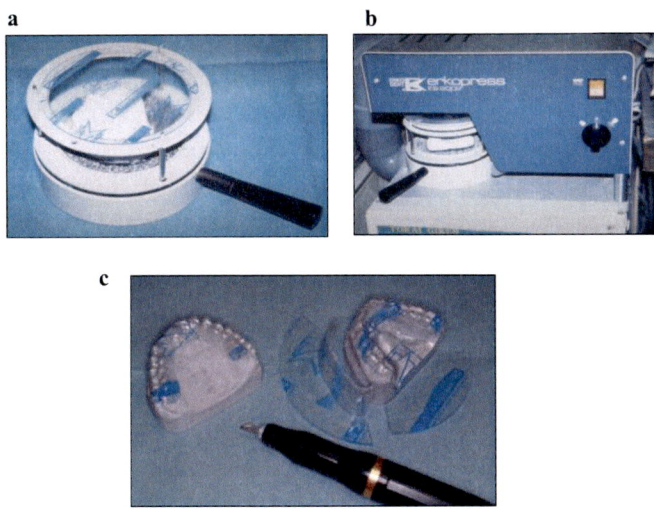

Figure 10. A copolyester foil was placed in the apparatus (a) and plasticized until the foil sagged downwards slightly and permanent impressions could be created by a blunt instrument (b). The foil was then molded. The desired outline of the splints was marked on the foil and cut using a twist drill (c).

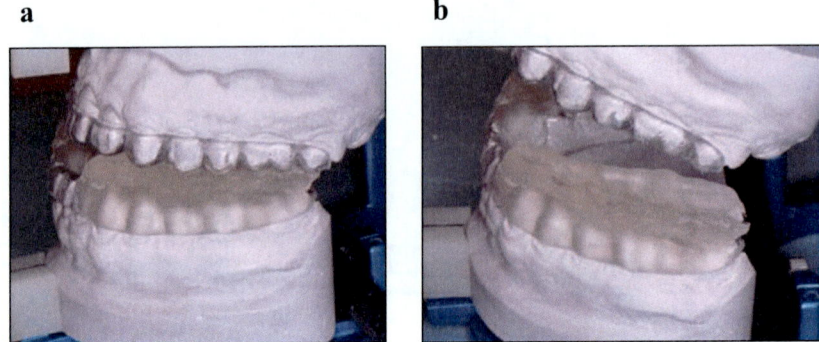

Figure 11. Rims were created with autopolymerizing resin in the mandibular, leaving a slight separation.

The cast undercuts are blocked out with wax (Modellier-Wax, Erkodent, Pfalzgrafenweiler, Germany) and duplicated. A copolyester foil (2 mm thick, 120 mm in diameter, Erkodur, Erkodent, Germany) is placed in the apparatus (Erkopress ES 2002, Erkodent, Germany) and plasticized until the foil sags downwards slightly and permanent impressions can be created by a blunt instrument. The foil is then molded. The desired outline of the splints is marked on the foil and cut using a twist drill (Figure 10). The master casts and splints are mounted in the articulator using the interocclusal record. Rims are created with autopolymerizing resin (Quick Resin, Shofu, Japan) in the mandibular, leaving a 1 mm separation (Figure 11). The buccal and lingual contours of the rims should be continuous. After checking for retentiveness of the maxillary and mandibular splints, they are attached together in the mouth of the patient with autopolymerizing resin (Quick Resin, Shofu, Japan). Then the device is polished and completed. This appliance enlarges the upper airway, inhibits mouth breathing and facilitates nasal breathing (Figure 5a, b). An anterior opening can be made if the patient finds it hard to insert the appliance because of nasal congestion (Figure 5c). The patient is instructed on how to insert and remove the appliances, as well as possible side effects that may occur the first morning after use, such as transient tooth, temporomandibular joint or muscle discomfort for a brief time after awakening. The device should be kept in water when it is not used. At the first follow-up appointment, normally after a week, the device is checked for retention and stability. If retention is insufficient, the device is rebased by means of the autopolymerizing resin. Where further additional retention is needed, wrought wire Adams or ball clasps are incorporated within the splints.

If the patient has muscle or temporomandibular joint discomfort, the appliance is separated and rejoined at a decreased protrusive position. This adjustment is repeated until all discomfort has disappeared.

a.1. Indications

The American Academy of Sleep Medicine has issued practice guidelines stating that oral appliance therapy is indicated for simple snoring and mild SAS, and for moderate to severe SAS if CPAP is not accepted or if surgery is inappropriate [33]. Although CPAP has a better therapeutic effect than oral appliance therapy, it is poorly tolerated and less used by many patients. Another indication of oral appliance therapy is upper airway resistance syndrome [44]. Upper airway resistance syndrome (UARS) is a form of sleep-disordered breathing in which repetitive increases in resistance to airflow within the upper airway lead to multiple, brief arousals and daytime hypersomnolence [45-47]. Many patients prefer an oral appliance if CPAP is poorly tolerated or the effect of surgery is inadequate [9]. In more than half of patients, an oral appliance is enough effective enough and they use only the oral appliance (Figure 12).

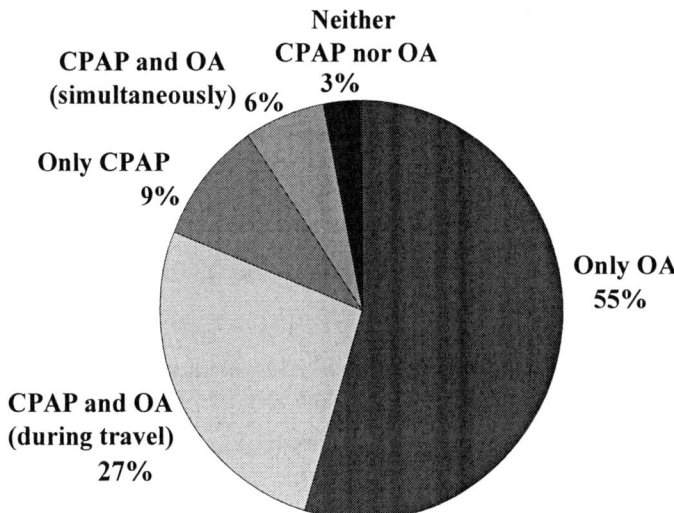

Figure 12. Final status of use in SAS patients (n=64) who experienced both CPAP and oral appliance (OA). In more than half of patients the oral appliance showed enough effectiveness and they used only the oral appliance. Some patients used CPAP daily and their oral appliance during business trip soar travel. Some other patients simultaneously used CPAP and their oral appliance.

Some patients use CPAP daily and an oral appliance during business trips or travel. Some other patients simultaneously use CPAP and an oral appliance, in which case, the mandible is maintained at a protrusive position and the pressure of CPAP can be minimal.

It is preferable for the patient to have enough teeth to adequately anchor the appliance. If dentures fit well, an oral appliance can be fabricated and inserted on the dentures for patients with fewer teeth. For edentulous patients a tongue retaining device can be applied (Figure 6a,b). In patients with temporomandibular joint disorders, particularly patients with myofacial pain, oral appliances should be carefully applied.

Some patients discontinue the appliance because of temporomandibular joint or masticatory muscle pain. However, other patients showed improvement of symptoms of temporomandibular joint disorders such as clicking. We often use a repositioning splint which advances the mandible to treat anterior disc derangement. Perhaps the oral appliance for SAS treatment functions equally and improves the temporomandibular joint sounds.

Abnormality or characteristics on cephalography of SAS patients are reported (Figure 13). Non-obese SAS patients, often observed in the Japanese population, tend to show skeletal abnormality, while obese SAS patients have a tendency toward abnormality of the soft tissue. Many patients show micrognathia or a tendency of retrognathia, macroglossia. The appliance is significantly effective for patients who exhibit a tendency toward micrognathia (Figure 14) or a short soft palate (Figure 15) [19].

However, since the appliance prevents the mandible from collapsing by advancing it, if other factors influence airway obstruction, the sleep apnea will not improve.

Narrowing or obstruction are influenced by functional and anatomic factors. Functional factors include respiratory instability, lax tissues surrounding the oropharynx, and deficient contraction of the pharyngeal dilator muscles [8]. Anatomic factors include abnormally narrow airways, thick and long velum palatinum, tonsillar and adenoid hypertrophy, micrognathia and retrognathia, nasal insufficiency, fat infiltration of the oropharynx, open mandibular angle, hypertrophy and thickness of the tongue, and lowered hyoid bone [8].

Cephalography is effective for indications and predictable criteria of an oral appliance. The anatomical factors in severe cases must be treated surgically; otorhynolaryngeal surgery or CPAP are considered if the obstruction is observed in multiple sites or the site covers a wide area. There is no reliable diagnostic method to predict the treatment outcome of oral appliance therapy. Further studies are necessary.

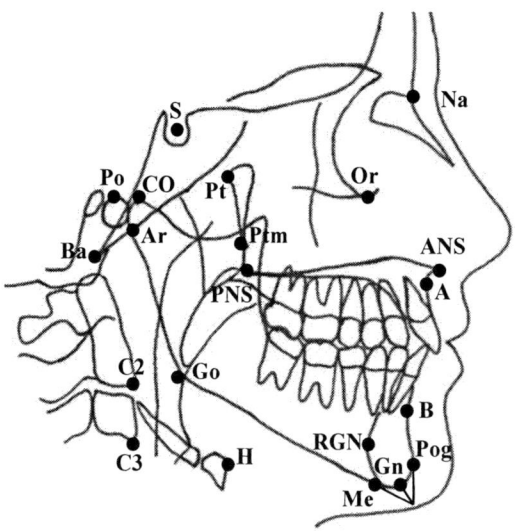

Figure 13. Reference points for cephalometric analysis for SAS patients. S: sella point, Ba: basion, Ar: articulare, Ptm: pterygomaxillare, Pt: pterygoid point, Po: porion, Na: nasion, ANS: anterior nasal spine, A: subspinale, Or: orbitale, PNS: posterior nasal spine, B: supramentale, Pog: pogonion, RGN: retrognathion, Me: menton, Go: gonion, Gn: gnathion, CO: condilion, H: hyoid bone, C2: the most antero-inferior point of the second vertebral corpus, C3: the most antero-inferior point of the third vertebral corpus.

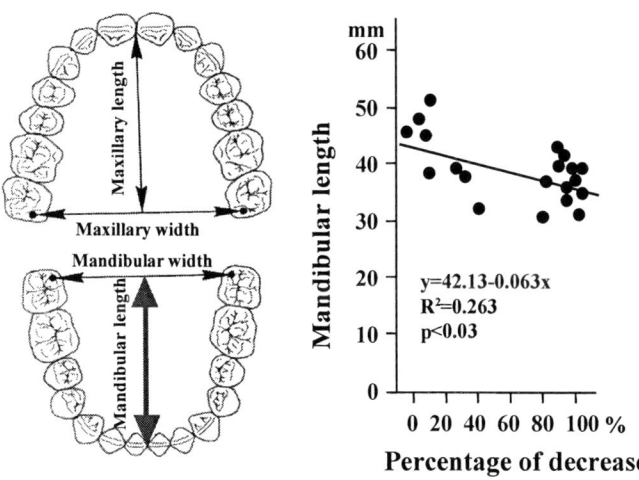

Figure 14. Correlation between mandibular length and percentage decrease of apnea index. Mandibular length decreased significantly (p<0.03) with the percentage decrease in the apnea index (n=20).

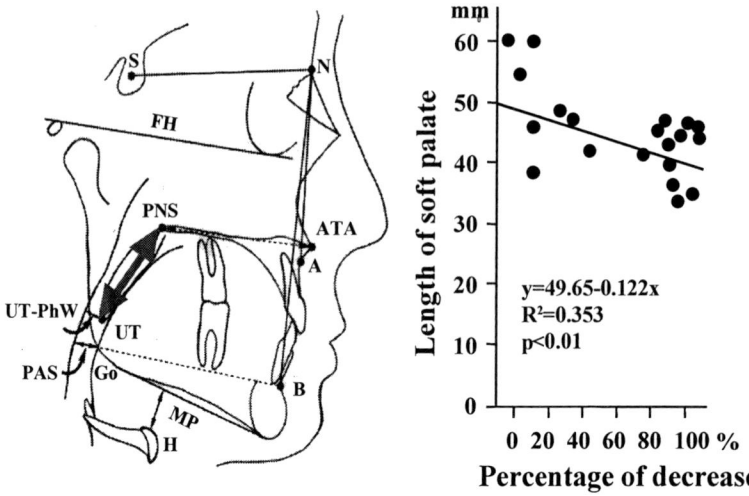

Figure 15. Correlation between length of the soft palate and percentage decrease of apnea index. The length of the soft palate was inversely correlated with the percentage of decrease (n=20). S: sella point, N: nasion, FH: Frankfort horizontal plane, PNS: posterior nasal spine, ATA: spinal point, A: subspinale, B: supramentale, UT: tip of uvula, UT-PhW: distance from UT to middle pharyngeal wall, PAS: posterior nasal spine, Go: gonion, MP: mandibular plane, H: hyoid bone.

a.2. Mechanism of Action of Oral Appliance

Oral appliances are thought to improve upper airway patency by advancing the mandible and/or tongue. This may lead to an improvement in upper airway dimensions and possible effects on upper airway muscle tone. Greater amounts of mandibular protrusion are associated with the ability of the appliance to reduce the AHI. These results indicate that increases in upper airway size at multiple levels by advancing the mandible are important in producing the clinical effects.

The differences of the effect of oral appliances on upper airway size are likely related to the differences in methodology. Mandibular advancement during general anesthesia can increase airway size in both the retropalatal and retroglossal area and reduce closing pressure [48]. The results of the effects of oral appliances on upper airway size using upright lateral cephalometry with films taken during wakefulness are sometimes conflicting; an oral appliance increased the majority of subjects in some studies [16, 49] but not in another study [50]. Other studies using upright lateral cephalometry showed that an oral appliance lowers the tongue position and reduce the mandibular plane to hyoid distance, advancing the mandible and widening the upper oropharynx (retropalatal and retroglossal) in some subjects [49, 51]. Using supine cephalograms, similar results in the mandibular plane to hyoid distance and in airway size and cross-sectional area have also been reported [52-54]. Other imaging modalities such as computed tomography and videoendoscopy have confirmed increases in pharyngeal airway size [49, 55, 56], volume [57] and cross-sectional area in the velopharynx [58]. These studies indicated increases in cross-sectional area of the velopharynx, in the lateral and anteroposterior dimensions, and high up in the oropharynx. Therefore the tongue, soft palate, lateral pharyngeal walls and mandible can interact to control airway size, and mandibular advancement may induce complex and variable changes in these structures.

Increased neuromuscular activity is another potential mechanism of action of oral appliances. In one study, muscle tone in the genioglossus, masseter and lateral pterygoid muscles was augmented following oral appliance insertion [59]. Another study also found an increase of genioglossus activity with mandibular advancement [60]. These studies suggest that mandibular advancement can activate the upper airway muscles and contribute airway patency. In two placebo controlled trials [61, 62], oral appliance without advancement as a control showed no clinical effect. Therefore, mandibular advancement is required for the oral appliance to improve SAS. Mandibular advancement might trigger stretch receptors which activate the upper airway muscles. The mode of action of the oral appliance is probably multifactorial, involving both a structural change with enhancement of the caliber of the upper airway as a result of mandibular protrusion, but also by triggering stretch receptors which activate the airway support muscles [63].

a.3. Effect of Oral Appliance

The author has treated over 2,000 patients with SAS and snoring using mainly oral appliances [9, 19, 22, 39]. The diagnosis of SAS was based on the combination of typical complaints such as loud and irregular snoring, daytime hypersomnolence, and polysomnographic findings. Patients were unselected apart from the following inclusion criteria: (1) present enough teeth to adequately anchor the appliance, (2) no arthralgia, myofacial pain or joint sounds due to temporomandibular joint disorders. Evaluation of each patient included a complete history, physical examination, and intraoral examination.

Standard all-night polysomnographic recordings were performed twice, with and without the device, using a computer (Medilog SAC 847 system, Oxford Instruments, England) as described previously [19, 22]. The recording with the device was performed after a habituation period (33 ± 13.5 days). The recordings included electroencephalograms, electrooculograms, submental electromyograms, electrocardiograms, nasal and oral airflow, thoracic and abdominal chest movement, finger oxymetry and body position [64]. The apnea, hypopnea and their type were determined. Apnea was defined as the cessation of airflow at the nose and mouth lasting for more than 10 s, while hypopnea was defined as a decrease of 50 % or more in thoracoabdominal motion associated with a fall in baseline oxygen saturation of 3 % or more. The minimum event length was 10 s, and mean and longest duration of event was recorded. The apnea-hypopnea index (AHI) and apnea index (AI) were calculated by dividing the total number of events by the sleep duration. Two criteria, a fall in the AHI to < 10 and a 50 % reduction in AHI were used to define treatment responders. Sleep efficiency was defined as the total sleep time divided by the time from sleep onset to final awaking in the morning. Two criteria, a fall in AHI to < 10 or 5 and a 50 % reduction in AHI were used to define treatment responders. Sleep stages were scored manually according to established criteria [64]. An arousal was defined as interruption of sleep by continuous alpha activity and increased electromyographic activity over 3 s. The arousal index was the mean number of arousals per hour.

a.3.1. AHI

Different criteria, such as a decrease in AHI to <10 or 20 [29, 65], and a reduction in the AHI by >50 % [20, 22] have been used to define treatment success. The success rate, defined as a reduction of AHI to less than 10, was 54 % in 2087 patients, and the response rate, defined as at least 50 % reduction in the AHI (although it still remained above 10), was 21 % in 1577 patients [32]. In this study, responders defined by AHI < 10 were 54 % and those defined as a 50 % fall of AHI were 61 %. Oral appliances reduced initial AHI by 42 %, CPAP reduced it by 75 %, and uvulopalatopharyngoplasty by 30 % [32]. In an early study by the author [22], 256 patients (33 women and 223 men) between 28 and 83 years of age [mean age 53.6 ± 8.9 (SD) years] were recruited. The patients were treated before 1994. The mean body mass index was $28.3 ± 2.8$ kg/m^2 (range 21 to 39 kg/m^2). Responders defined by AHI < 10 were 138 out of 256 patients (54.0 %). Responders defined as a 50 % reduction in AHI were 169 patients (66.0 %). Table 1 presents a summary of the sleep data for pretreatment and posttreatment polysomnographic recordings. The mean AHI was 25.8 ± 18.2 (SD), and this decreased significantly (p<0.0001, t-test) after insertion of the device (12.0 ± 12.8). The mean AI, obstructive AI, and mixed AI were decreased significantly with the device, while central AI was increased slightly but not significantly (Table 1).

Table 1. Respiratory function variables with and without the appliance

	Baseline		Treatment		
	Mean ± SD	Range	Mean ± SD	Range	P value
Apnea-hypopnea index (AHI)(No./h)	43.2 ± 25.2	1.2-89.8	18.2 ± 21.3	0.0-75.3	0.0001
Obstructive AHI (No./h)	25.6 ± 18.1	0.0-57.6	8.0 ± 12.1	0.0-53.6	0.0001
Central AHI (No./h)	1.6 ± 2.1	0.0-9.2	1.8 ± 2.6	0.0-7.8	NS
Mixed AHI (No./h)	16.1 ± 18.2	0.0-58.1	8.4 ± 12.5	0.0-58.0	0.005
Apnea index (AI)(No./h)	25.8 ± 18.2	0.0-75.2	12.0 ± 12.8	0.0-69.8	0.0001
Obstructive AI (No./h)	11.2 ± 12.6	0.0-51.5	6.6 ± 8.8	0.0-30.4	0.005
Central AI (No./h)	1.3 ± 1.5	0.0-6.4	1.6 ± 1.9	0.0-7.7	NS
Mixed AI (No./h)	13.3 ± 11.6	0.0-42.5	4.0 ± 8.9	0.0-33.0	0.0001
Mean apnea duration (s)	23.8 ± 5.7	12.0-34.1	19.3 ± 5.6	11.3-30.8	0.0001
Longest apnea duration (s)	59.2 ± 32.3	14.0-153.5	44.6 ± 21.0	13.0-83.0	0.0005
Mean oxgen saturation (%)	92.1 ± 2.5	81.0-95.0	93.3 ± 2.0	84.0-96.3	0.0005
Minimal oxygen saturation (%)	72.6 ± 9.2	51.0-89.0	75.2 ± 8.3	52.0-86.3	0.05

NS: not significant.

Mean and longest apnea duration were reduced significantly (Table 1). The mean and minimal oxygen saturation was significantly higher with than without the appliance. In a recent study by the author [66], responders defined by AHI < 5 were more than 60 % and those defined as a 50 % fall of AHI were 80 %. The mean AHI of all patients (17.9±14.1) was significantly ($p<0.001$) decreased after oral appliance therapy (5.8±5.9). Mean AHI reduction in all the patients was 67.6%; 58.8% of the patients achieved a complete response (AHI<5), 21.6% had a partial response (AHI reduction ≧50%, but AHI≧5), and 19.6% were classed as treatment failure (AHI reduction <50%). Responders defined as a 50 % fall of AHI were 80.4 %.

a.3.2. Sleep Quality Variables

Normal sleep is characterized by 2 to 5 % of stage 1 sleep, 45 to 55 % of stage 2 sleep, 13 to 23 % of slow-wave sleep, and 20 to 25 % of rapid eye movement sleep in young adults [67]. The changes in sleep structure in the current study were in the direction of improvement with the appliance. Sleep quality variables with and without the oral appliance are listed in Table 2. The total sleep time and proportion of sleep time in each sleep position did not differ significantly between the two recording sessions.

Table 2. Sleep quality variables with and without the appliance

	Baseline		Treatment		
	Mean ± SD	Range	Mean ± SD	Range	P value
Total sleep time (min)	430.5 ± 102.6	165.5-567.0	449.3 ± 72.0	335.2-561.5	NS
Sleep efficiency (%)	84.2 ± 13.6	36.7-99.6	85.8 ± 9.8	64.7-99.6	0.05
Stage 1 sleep (%)	18.8 ± 9.9	5.1-52.6	15.5 ± 9.5	3.3-38.5	0.005
Stage 2 sleep (%)	46.1 ± 13.6	22.2-76.5	45.3 ± 13.6	19.6-71.9	NS
Stage 3 sleep (%)	6.8 ± 8.2	0.0-33.8	6.4 ± 2.7	1.0-13.2	NS
Stage 4 sleep (%)	3.7 ± 6.7	0.0-20.9	3.7 ± 5.8	0.0-20.5	NS
Rapid eye movement sleep (%)	9.1 ± 8.3	0.0-27.8	13.6 ± 4.2	7.2-26.8	0.05
Total arousal (No.)	94.9 ± 85.6	25-422	67.8 ± 46.9	2-223	0.05

NS: not significant.

The changes in sleep structure were in the direction of improvement with the appliance. Stage 1 sleep decreased from 19 % to 16 % (p<0.005), and rapid eye movement sleep increased from 9 % to 14 % (p<0.05). Sleep efficiency improved significantly. Total arousal was reduced significantly (p<0.05) after insertion of the device from 95 to 68.

a.3.3. Sleepiness

Excessive daytime sleepiness with SAS has public health implications. Epidemiological evidence suggests that SAS is linked to the symptom of excessive daytime sleepiness. The most common single way of assessing subjective daytime function is the Epworth Sleepiness Scale (ESS). In previous studies, the ESS dropped with oral appliance use. In 19 investigations, in which data used in calculation, there was a significant reduction in the ESS from 11.2 to 7.8. Use of oral appliances improves daytime function; the ESS dropped from 11.2 to 7.8 (-3.4 units) in 854 patients in a recent review [32]. CPAP showed significant improvement of ESS (parallel-group studies: -3.83 units, crossover studies: -1.84 units) [68].

The effect of oral appliances on objective excessive daytime sleepiness remains uncertain. Some investigations reported improvements in vigilance test, maintenance of wakefulness test, and multiple sleep latency test. Findings from comparisons of oral appliances with other treatments such as CPAP in the response of subjective excessive daytime sleepiness have been divergent. Oral appliances improve excessive daytime sleepiness, but are not necessarily superior or consistently preferred to other treatments. ESS improved significantly after insertion of the appliance (Table 2).

a.3.4. Snoring

Snoring is a sound produced by the vibrating structure of the upper airway. Although snoring is the cardinal symptom of SAS, the difficulties with its definition are the reasons why objective measurement of sound is seldom a routine part of polysomnography. Recent randomized controlled trials of oral appliances in SAS revealed that both snoring frequency and intensity are significantly reduced compared to no treatment and a control appliance. The mean reduction in snoring with oral appliance therapy was 45 % based on pooled data in 18 studies involving 529 patients [32]. However, there are many causes for snoring. If the real reason is the nasopharynx, treatment by an otorynolaryngologist is necessary.

a.3.5. Blood Pressure

SAS has been identified as an independent risk factor for arterial hypertension [69, 70]. Studies on the specific effects of SAS treatment on blood pressure are confusing. Uncontrolled studies reported that mean arterial blood pressure substantially decreased with effective CPAP [71-73], while randomized controlled trials of CPAP treatment on blood pressure in SAS showed either no effect [74-76], a limited decrease in blood pressure by 1.4 mmHg [77] and 2.5 mmHg [78], or a substantial reduction by 10 mmHg [79]. A recent controlled study of oral appliance treatment revealed a significant fall in blood pressure by approximately 3 mmHg [80], while two studies comparing CPAP and oral appliance therapy reported a significant improvement in nighttime diastolic blood pressure by 2 mmHg for the latter technique [76] and 2mmHg reduction with oral appliance and 5.1 mmHg fall with CPAP [81].

The authors studied 161 patients [121 men and 40 women, mean age 54.3 ± 13.7 (SD) years, body mass index (BMI); 24.9 ± 4.2] diagnosed with SAS [mean apnea-hypopnea index (AHI); 17.9 ± 14.1] [66]. Patient characteristics are summarized in Table 3. Eighty-one patients (51.2%) were hypertensive (systolic blood pressure≧140mmHg and/or diastolic blood pressure≧90mmHg) with 51 of them on antihypertensive medication.

Systolic, diastolic and mean blood pressure plus heart rate were recorded at rest and repeated in a sitting position using an automatic blood pressure monitor (BP-203RVII, Colin, Japan) between 9:00 and 11:00 am. The measurement was repeated at least twice on one day. If the values showed a significant large fluctuation, the third or fourth measurement was carried out after an interval of several minutes. The averaged values were recorded as the blood pressure of that day. Before treatment, the measurements were performed at least twice and the mean value defined as blood pressure before treatment. The measurement was conducted on every follow-up visit and mean values of the two or three days following appliance insertion were defined as blood pressure after treatment. Mean values at approximately 60 day intervals after insertion of the appliance were recorded.

Individual customized appliances (Figure 5) were fabricated. The sleep study was performed in hospital according to standard criteria. Each patient was studied before and after insertion of the oral appliance after a suitable habituation period which averaged 60 days. The patients were subdivided into three groups; responder, partial responder and nonresponder groups, according to the change of the recorded mean arterial pressure fall.

Patients used their appliances for a mean duration of 6.9±1.3 hours each night. Table 3 presents a summary of blood pressure and sleep data with and without the oral appliance in place. The mean AHI of all patients (17.9±14.1, range; 5-67.5) was significantly (p<0.001) decreased after oral appliance therapy (5.8±5.9, range;0.4-33.8). Mean AHI reduction in all the patients was 67.6%; 58.8% of the patients achieved a complete response (AHI<5), 21.6% had a partial response (AHI reduction ≧ 50%, but AHI ≧ 5), and 19.6% were classed as treatment failure (AHI reduction <50%). The other respiratory and sleep variables such as mean and minimal oxygen saturation, arousal index and ESS improved significantly (Table 4). There was no relevant change in body weight of the patients.

The systolic (132.0±16.1mmHg) and diastolic (82.1±10.6mmHg) blood pressure were significantly (p<0.001) reduced after treatment (127.5±15.0mmHg, 79.2±10.0mmHg, respectively). The mean arterial pressure (107.1±12.9mmHg) showed a significant (p<0.001) fall (103.4±12.0mmHg). Oral appliance therapy produced drops in systolic (by 4.5±7.4mmHg), diastolic (by 3.0±6.3mmHg) and mean arterial (by 3.7±6.1mmHg) blood pressure. The heart rate was slightly, but not significantly reduced.

Table 3. Respiratory and sleep variables and blood pressure at baseline and on treatment.

	Baseline		Treatment		
	Mean ± SD	Range	Mean ± SD	Range	P value
Blood pressure variables					
Systolic blood pressure (mmHg)	132.0 ± 16.1	89 - 178	127.5 ± 15.0	94 - 167	0.001
Diastolic blood pressure (mmHg)	82.1 ± 10.6	55 - 118	79.2 ± 10.0	57 - 108	0.001
Mean blood pressure (mmHg)	107.1 ± 12.9	72 - 148	103.4 ± 12.0	76.5 - 137.5	0.001
Heart rate (bpm)	73.3 ± 12.5	47 - 115	73.2 ± 12.1	50 - 114	NS
Respiratory and sleep variables					
Apnea-hypopnea index (No./h)	17.9 ± 14.1	5 - 67.5	5.8 ± 5.9	0.4 - 33.8	0.001
Mean oxygen saturation (%)	95.4 ± 1.8	84 - 99	95.9 ± 1.5	91 - 99	0.05
Minimal oxygen saturation (%)	79.3 ± 8.3	51 - 92	85.0 ± 5.9	62 - 94	0.001
Arousal index (No./h)	29.5 ± 14.7	8.1 - 73.1	16.2 ± 6.8	0.9 - 24.8	0.05
Epworth Sleepiness Scale	7.1 ± 3.9	0 - 18	4.1 ± 2.7	0 - 12	0.0001

The respiratory and sleep variables improved significantly (n=161). The systolic, diastolic and mean blood pressure were significantly (p<0.001) reduced after treatment. The mean arterial pressure response was significantly correlated with baseline blood pressure and with AHI reduction (p<0.05).

The mean arterial pressure response was significantly correlated with baseline blood pressure (systolic: r=0.33, p<0.001, diastolic: r=0.4, p<0.001, mean: r=0.37, p<0.001) and with AHI reduction (r=0.29, p<0.05). There were no other significant correlations between the blood pressure response and other variables.

The patients were subdivided into responders, partial responders, and nonresponders based on the averaged mean arterial pressure fall (3.7mmHg) after treatment. Characteristics in the mean arterial pressure responders (fall>3.7 mmHg), the partial responders (0<fall≦3.7mmHg) and the nonresponders (fall≦ 0mmHg) are summarized in Table 4.

Table 4. Comparison of mean arterial pressure responders (fall>3.7mmHg), partial responders (0<fall≦3.7mmHg) and nonresponders (fall≦0mmHg)

	Responder (n=70)	Partial Responder (n=46)	Nonresponder (n=45)
Characteristics			
Sex, male:female	47:23	36:10	38:7
Age (y)	56.0 ± 12.6	52.0 ± 14.4	54.0 ± 14.6
Body mass index (kg/m^2)	24.8 ± 3.9	24.9 ± 4.9	24.8 ± 3.8
Disease duration (month)	129.7 ± 108.6	152.6 ± 145.8	164.9 ± 128.6
Hypertension (n)	39/70	21/46	21/31
Antihypertensive drug (n)	22/70	15/46	14/31
Blood pressure variables			
Systolic blood pressure (mmHg)	135.8 ± 16.7	131.7 ± 14.0	126.5 ± 16.0
SBP change (mmHg)	-10.5 ± 5.7	-2.8 ± 3.6	3.1 ± 3.9
Diastolic blood pressure (mmHg)	85.6 ± 10.6	80.6 ± 9.4	78.2 ± 10.3
DBP change (mmHg)	-8.2 ± 4.7	-1.1 ± 3.2	3.1 ± 3.7
Mean blood pressure (mmHg)	110.7 ± 13.1	106.2 ± 10.9	102.3 ± 12.8
MBP change (mmHg)	-9.3 ± 4.3	-2.0 ± 1.1	3.1 ± 2.5
Heart rate (bpm)	72.7 ± 11.7	74.0 ± 14.2	73.6 ± 12.1
Respiratory and sleep variables			
Apnea-hypopnea index (No./h)	16.4 ± 14.1	21.2 ± 15.5	17.0 ± 12.3
AHI reduction (%)	69.6 ± 17.9	65.9 ± 28.6	52.2 ± 28.4
Mean oxygen saturation (%)	95.4 ± 2.1	95.2 ± 1.5	95.6 ± 1.4)
Minimal oxygen saturation (%)	80.0 ± 7.0	76.3 ± 9.4	81.2 ± 8.5)
Arousal index (No./h)	30.1 ± 14.8	24.7 ± 14.1	34.8 ± 15.1
Epworth Sleepiness Scale	7.1 ± 3.7	7.1 ± 4.5	7.0 ± 3.5)

The three groups did not differ significantly in distribution of sex, hypertension, or use of antihypertensive drugs. Disease duration was longer in the nonresponders than in the responders, but not significantly so (p=0.08). The mean AHI reductions in the responders (69.6%) and the partial responders (65.9%) were significantly (p<0.05, ANOVA) higher than that in the nonresponders (52.2%). There were no significant differences in any of the variables except blood pressure between the three groups at baseline.

This study demonstrated that the selected and treated SAS patients showed a significant mean arterial pressure reduction by about 3.7 mmHg after oral appliance therapy. The response was correlated to baseline blood pressure and AHI reduction. It is therefore tempting to predict a reduction in the risk of stroke by 20 %, if 3 mm Hg blood pressure reduction were maintained for 2 to 3 years [82]. A mean blood pressure drop by 10 mmHg is estimated to reduce coronary heart disease event risk by 37 % and stroke risk by 56 % [82]. The blood pressure fall with oral appliance was observed to be most apparent in the early morning, which is the time of peak risk of acute myocardial infarction [83] and stroke [84]. In fact, a drop in blood pressure at this time of the day is suggested to provide further protection against these adverse cardiovascular events [80]. In this study the mean arterial blood pressure response was significantly correlated with baseline blood pressure recordings. Therefore, the magnitude and timing of an oral appliance's blood pressure lowering effect appears to be particularly beneficial for hypertensive patients with SAS, diminishing the excessive cardiovascular morbidity and mortality previously observed in SAS.

Although the precise mechanisms remain uncertain, the persistent increase in sympathetic activity caused by chronic apnea-associated repetitive asphyxia and arousal is thought to be the key mechanism in the pathogenesis of daytime arterial hypertension in patients with SAS [85]. The severity of SAS appears to be independently associated with systemic hypertension in a linear fashion [86], with the treatment of hypertensive subjects with SAS using CPAP resulting in an improvement in blood pressure readings [72, 77]. Randomized controlled trials of CPAP treatment on blood pressure in SAS showed either no effect [74-76], or only a limited decrease in blood pressure by 1.4 mmHg [77] and 2.5 mmHg [78], or else a substantial reduction by 10 mmHg [79]. A recent controlled study of oral appliance treatment revealed a significant drop in blood pressure by approximately 3 mmHg [80], while a placebo controlled study comparing the effectiveness of CPAP and oral appliance therapy reported a significant but limited improvement in nighttime diastolic blood pressure of 2 mmHg only with the oral appliance [76]. The response of such SAS treatment on high blood pressure would be influenced by baseline blood pressure and disease severity, treatment duration or effect, and the method of blood pressure measurement.

Both this study and other trials [79, 80] did not exclude patients who were hypertensive or taking antihypertensive medication. About 50 % of patients with SAS have daytime hypertension [87], and in this study 51 % of the patients were indeed hypertensive. The large number of patients in this study included a wide range of normotensive and hypertensive patients with mild to moderate SAS and who were generally identified as candidates for oral appliance therapy. The results of this study may therefore be generalized to the broad and typical SAS clinic population. This does not appears to be the case for a study [77] where hypertensive patients were excluded, or else reported to be less prevalent in the other reports [74-76]. The observed lack of effect or only minor decrease in blood pressure in these studies may account for a possible floor effect. The mean arterial pressure response was significantly correlated with baseline blood pressure in this study.

Although CPAP has a better therapeutic effect than oral appliance therapy, it is poorly tolerated and less used by many patients. The patients in this study used the oral appliance 6.9 hours per night and compared to 6.4 hours [81], 6.8 hours [80] and 5.5 hours [76] in other studies. On the other hand, reported CPAP compliance was 3.3 hours [77], 4.9 hours [78], 5.5 hours [79], 3.6 hours [76] and 4.2 hours [81]. A partial benefit of an oral appliance on sleep-disordered breathing sustained over a longer period of the night appears to be a similar blood pressure-lowering effect. Oral appliance therapy may very well be an important alternative to CPAP treatment in a significant number of patients, and can be prescribed for patients on CPAP treatment with low compliance.

A recent report revealed that oral appliance therapy significantly reduced systolic blood pressure by 3.3 mmHg and diastolic blood pressure by 3.4 mmHg [80]. On the other hand, another trial revealed that only nighttime diastolic pressure decreased significantly by 2.2 mmHg [76] and 2 mmHg [81]. In the present study, the patients showed a 3.7 mmHg reduction in mean arterial pressure and 4.7 mmHg fall [88] which may be related to the differences in intervention period and reduction in AHI with the appliance. The mean AHI reduction was 50 % [80], 34 % [76] and 49 % [81], but 67 % in this study, and elsewhere 75 % [88]. The mean arterial pressure response was significantly correlated with AHI reduction in this study and the results underscore the importance of highly effective treatment for reducing blood pressure.

Additionally, a 50 % reduction of AHI with subtherapeutic control CPAP resulted in a slight increase in blood pressure [79], while oral appliance therapy led to a significant fall in blood pressure (approximately 3 mmHg), although the patients had only a 50 % reduction in AHI [80]. The significant blood pressure reduction in oral appliance therapy may be influenced not only by AHI reduction in but also by other factors. The mode of action of the oral appliance is probably multifactorial, involving both a structural change with enhancement of the caliber of the upper airway as a result of mandibular protrusion and also a triggering of stretch receptors which activate the airway support muscles [63]. Hypotonia of the masticatory and tongue muscles and the weight of the mandible, particularly in the supine position, can lead to opening of the mouth, with further dorsal displacement of the mandible and tongue base. This results in pharyngeal narrowing and airway resistance, and ultimately, obstructive sleep apnea [59, 89]. The oral appliance helps to maintain the tonus of the muscles by protracting the tongue and mandible even during sleep at a protrusive position, which suggests that the activated muscles prevent the upper airway from collapsing [59, 89]. The mechanism by which oral appliance treatment reduces blood pressure may very well differ from that induced by CPAP treatment.

a.2.6. Upper Airway Resistance Syndrome

Upper airway resistance syndrome (UARS) is a form of sleep-disordered breathing in which repetitive increases in resistance to airflow within the upper airway lead to multiple brief arousals and daytime hypersomnolence [45-47]. Hypertension is an important sequela of this order, likely resulting from autonomic and cardiovascular changes induced by negative intrathoracic pressure. A definitive diagnosis of UARS is made when nocturnal esophageal pressure monitoring demonstrates crescendo changes in intrathoracic pressures followed by frequent arousals or microarousals [45].

CPAP can be applied as the most efficacious form of therapy, but, low patient compliance may limit its practical use [47]. The safety and efficacy of surgical treatments remain to be elucidated. Patients with UARS were treated by oral appliance, to evaluate its effect on respiratory function and sleep quality variables.

Thirty-two patients (15 women and 17 men) with UARS, between the ages of 28 and 49 [mean age 38.4 ± 6.4 (SD) years] were selected for the present study. The UARS diagnosis was made based on the combination of clinical complaints such as daytime hypersomnolence and fatigue, snoring, and polysomnographic findings [47]. Excessive daytime sleepiness was evaluated by the ESS [90]. Inclusion criteria were: (1) AHI<5, (2) ESS scores of >10, (3) arousal index>10. Mean body mass index was 25.2 ± 2.6 kg/m^2. The devices (Figure 5) were fabricated individually for each patient.

All patients underwent standard overnight polysomnography for two nights, before and after insertion of the device. The second recording with the device was conducted after a habituation period (14-60 days after first use of appliance). The morning after each overnight study, the patients had a multiple sleep latency test (MSLT) in accordance with published guidelines [91]. Snoring was estimated by a bedroom partner according to a four-grade questionnaire: "satisfactory effect", "slight effect", "no effect", or "worsened effect". Ten of the 32 patients did not snore.

The statistical significance of the change in the results before and after insertion of the device was assessed by the paired t-test.

ESS decreased significantly ($p<0.0001$, paired t-test) from 13.2 ± 1.3 before treatment to 5.8 ± 1.1 with the device. The mean MSLT score increased significantly ($p<0.0005$) from 6.3 ± 3.3 m to 12.9 ± 6.9 m. Snoring was satisfactorily reduced in all 22 snorers, as estimated by a bedroom partner.

Initially, the mean AHI was 3.1 ± 2.0, which decreased significantly (p<0.0001) after insertion of the device (1.9 ± 1.8). The minimal oxygen saturation was significantly higher with than without the appliance. The changes in sleep structure were in the direction of improvement with the appliance. Wake time decreased from 9.7 ± 3.9 % to 6.4 ± 2.6 % (p<0.005), and rapid eye movement sleep increased from 15.2 ± 4.1 % to 21.6 ± 3.4 % (p<0.0001). Sleep efficiency improved significantly (p<0.005). Total arousal index was reduced significantly (p<0.0001) after insertion of the device from 35.5 ± 8.8 to 8.9 ± 4.1. The mean length of follow-up was 25.5 ± 3.7 months. All the patients continued to wear the device.

Factors preventing the widespread use of nocturnal esophageal pressure monitoring for the definitive diagnosis of UARS include patient refusal or intolerance and the requirement of additional technical expertise and expense [92]. Therefore, many patients are diagnosed as having UARS, without esophageal pressure monitoring, on the basis of the qualitative perception of possible respiratory-related arousals from standard nocturnal polysomnography [47]. In the present study, the patients were diagnosed having UARS based on clinical inclusion criteria, as described previously [93]. Oral appliances are constructed with the goal of moving the position of the mandible and tongue forward to minimize the possibility of oropharyngeal obstruction. Patients with UARS presented a narrow posterior airway space behind the base of the tongue [46]. Hypotonia of the masticatory and tongue muscles and the weight of the mandible, particularly in the supine position, can lead to passive mouth opening and further dorsal displacement of the mandible and tongue, resulting in pharyngeal narrowing and airway resistance [59, 89]. The appliance is suggested to maintain the activity of the muscles protracting the tongue and mandible at an increased vertical and protrusive position [59, 89]. As a result, repeated increases in resistance to airflow within the upper airway seemed to be reduced, resulting in significant reductions of arousal and excessive daytime sleepiness in this study. Based on its effectiveness and good compliance, the oral appliance is an important treatment choice and may be the preferred initial treatment for UARS.

a.3.7. Side Effects

The more protrusive the mandibular position, the more patent the upper airway, and the better the effect. Nevertheless, the maximal protrusive position can cause discomfort of the temporomandibular joint or masticatory muscles, resulting in pain, and possibly in craniomandibular disorder. The most suitable mandible position must be individual for each patient. The final protrusion distance represents a delicate balance between side effects and efficacy.

Therefore, the fabrication and fitting of the appliance should be done by a dentist with expertise in this area. Side effects of masticatory muscles or temporomandibular joint for a brief time after awakening are sometimes reported by patients just after initial use of the appliance. With regular use, adjustment and possibly rejoining splints after separation, these symptoms normally subside. In principle, the patients should insert the device during sleep for life and must be free of myofacial or temporomandibular joint symptoms and changes in occlusal alignment. Therefore, the device should offer full occlusal coverage to prevent vertical changes to the dentition over time. Side effects were transitory and tolerable.

Common side effects include temporomandibular joint pain, myofacial pain, tooth pain, salivation, temporomandibular joint sounds, dry mouth and morning-after occlusal changes [9, 22, 39]. It is also reported that minor tooth movement and small changes in the occlusion developed in some patients after prolonged use [94, 95].

In a previous study with a mean length of follow-up of 30.5 months [22], 22 of 256 patients (8.6 %) experienced transitory discomfort of masticatory muscles or temporomandibular joint a few days after the first use of the device. However, in most cases the discomfort disappeared spontaneously after several days. Five patients (2 %) discontinued the appliance because of discomfort of the temporomandibular joint or masticatory muscles. Side effects were minor and tolerable, and no serious complications were observed. Eighteen patients (7 %) underwent CPAP or surgery because of unsuccessful efficacy with the device. Compliance with this appliance was 90.1 % (232 patients).

a.4. Factors Influencing the Effect

Appliances have not always led to sufficient improvement. The reasons for failures are complicated and are related to the different complications of skeletal, soft tissue, and functional aspects that produce upper airway obstruction in each patient. There is still a lively debate as to the relative contributions of abnormal anatomy and physiology in the pathogenesis of upper airway obstruction during sleep.

a.4.1. Anatomical Factors

The most common sites of airway obstruction are thought to be behind the base of the tongue (retroglossal) and behind the soft palate (retropalatal). The appliance is significantly effective for patients who exhibit a tendency toward micrognathia and a short soft palate (Figures 14, 15) [19]. Since the appliance prevents the mandible from collapsing by advancing it, if other factors influence airway obstruction, the sleep apnea will not improve. Narrowing or obstruction are influenced by functional and anatomic factors. Anatomic factors include abnormally narrow airways, thick and long velum palatinum, tonsillar and adenoid hypertrophy, micrognathia and retrognathia, nasal insufficiency, fat infiltration of the oropharynx, open mandibular angle, hypertrophy and thickness of the tongue, and lowered hyoid bone [8].

a.4.2. Functional Factors

Functional factors include respiratory instability, lax tissues surrounding the oropharynx, and deficient contraction of the pharyngeal dilator muscles [8]. The device is successful for obstructive and mixed apneas, but not suitable for central apnea [21, 59], which can occur upon loss of neural chest and abdominal respiratory drive even if the muscles are active and the upper airway is patent. Oral appliances appear to be less effective when the respiratory disturbance index exceeds 40 to 50 per hour, or AHI of > 60 [65]. A recent study reported that the success rate of oral appliance therapy correlated inversely to disease severity [20]. The reasons for the poor beneficial effect in severe cases remain unresolved.

a.4.3. Sleep Position

Snorers have long been recognized to snore most loudly while sleeping in the supine position [96]. When apnea patients sleep in the supine position there is a tendency for the tongue to relapse against the pharyngeal wall and, furthermore, during rapid eye movement sleep, with the additional factors of reduced tone in the genioglossal muscle, apneas are more frequent and prolonged than when patients sleep in a semiprone position [96]. Clinical use of the oral appliance is spreading, but sufficient improvement has not been attained in all patients. The reasons for failure are complicated because the upper airway obstruction results from combinations of disproportionate skeletal and soft tissue anatomy and functional factors. It is likely that oral appliance therapy is influenced by the sleep posture. Thus, the influence of sleep position on the efficacy of oral appliance therapy was evaluated polysomnographically before and after insertion of the device.

Seventy-two patients (10 women and 62 men) between 37 and 72 years of age [mean age 53.3 ± 9.2 (SD) years] with SAS were recruited [97]. The body mass index was between 21 and 39 kg/m^2 with a mean of 27.9 ± 2.9 kg/m^2. An appliance (Figure 5) was fabricated individually for each patient. After the habituation period, another polysomnographic evaluation was performed to assess the efficacy.

Standard all-night polysomnographic recordings were performed twice, before and after insertion of the device. The period between the two recordings was 36 ± 14.2 days. The recordings included body position using a body position sensor (BP-90C-088M, Oxford Instruments).

Sleep position was continuously monitored throughout the night on a TV monitor in the control room and recorded on a video camera. The patients were classified into three groups; supine, lateral and prone groups, according to the position in which the apneas and hypopneas were most frequently observed before treatment.

Table 5 shows the mean pretreatment and posttreatment polysomnographic values. The mean AHI was decreased significantly ($p<0.0001$, t-test) from 43.0 ± 25.6 before treatment to 21.6 ± 18.3 after insertion of the device. Responders defined by AHI < 10 were 38 out of 72 patients (52.8 %).

Responders defined as a 50 % reduction in AHI were 44 patients (61.1 %). Of the total sleep apneas, 70.8 %, 22.0 %, and 7.2 %, occurred in the supine, lateral and prone positions, respectively. In the supine position AHI decreased significantly from 29.8 ± 26.1 before treatment to 11.3 ± 13.8 with the appliance (Figure 16).

In the prone position AHI also showed a significant decrease from 5.5 ± 8.6 to 1.6 ± 2.9 without the device (Figure 16). In contrast, in the lateral position AHI increased slightly, but not significantly, from 7.7 ± 11.8 to 8.7 ± 12.0 after treatment.

Total AI, obstructive AI and mixed AI were decreased significantly with the device, while central AI increased slightly, but not significantly (Table 6, Figure 17). The mean and longest apnea duration were reduced significantly (Table 6). The mean and minimal oxygen saturation were significantly higher with than without the appliance.

Sleep quality variables with and without the oral appliance are listed in Table 6. Total sleep time and proportion of sleep time in each sleep position did not differ significantly between the two recording occasions. The sleep structure showed improvement after insertion of the appliance. Stage 1 sleep was decreased significantly, and rapid eye movement sleep was increased significantly. Sleep efficiency was improved from 85.1 ± 12.9 % to 90.5 ± 6.8 %, but not significantly ($p=0.03$).

Arousal indices were reduced after insertion of the device, but not significantly (Table 6).

Table 5. The results of sleep study in all 72 patients with and without the appliance

	Pretreatment		Posttreatment		
	Mean ± SD	Range	Mean ± SD	Range	P value
Respiratory function variables					
Apnea-hypopnea index (No./h)	43.0 ± 25.6	6.4 - 89.8	21.6 ± 18.3	1.8 - 75.3	0.0001
Apnea index (No./h)	25.6 ± 19.8	2.0 - 75.2	11.5 ± 13.8	0.4 - 69.8	0.0001
Mean event duration (s)	23.3 ± 5.6	14.0 - 34.9	21.2 ± 5.2	14.0 - 31.0	0.0001
Longest event duration (s)	77.8 ± 37.9	26.0 - 159.0	64.2 ± 21.6	31.0 - 99.0	0.0001
Mean oxgen saturation (%)	92.2 ± 2.7	81.0 - 95.0	93.3 ± 2.0	84.0 - 96.0	0.0001
Minimal oxygen saturation (%)	72.3 ± 10.6	51.0 - 89.0	75.3 ± 8.3	52.0 - 86.0	0.0041
Sleep quality variables					
Total sleep time (min)	434.3 ± 102.8	165.5 - 567.0	458.5 ± 67.7	335.5 - 561.5	0.8314
Supine sleep (%)	58.2 ± 37.5	0 – 100	44.9 ± 40.2	0 - 100	0.3115
Lateral sleep (%)	19.9 ± 20.6	0 - 55.5	26.1 ± 32.6	0 - 93.0	0.1721
Prone sleep (%)	21.9 ± 37.8	0 – 100	28.0 ± 43.2	0 - 100	0.8750
Stage 1 sleep (%)	19.3 ± 11.3	5.1 - 52.6	14.4 ± 7.5	3.3 - 37.8	0.0001
Stage 2 sleep (%)	46.0 ± 14.0	22.2 - 76.5	45.5 ± 15.1	19.6 - 71.9	0.0530
Stage 3 sleep (%)	6.8 ± 8.3	0.0 - 33.8	6.4 ± 2.9	1.0 - 11.4	0.8462
Stage 4 sleep (%)	3.7 ± 7.0	0.0 - 20.9	3.6 ± 5.8	0.0 - 20.3	0.0720
Rapid eye movement sleep (%)	9.3 ± 8.5	0.0 - 27.8	14.5 ± 5.2	7.2 - 24.6	0.0003
Arousal index (No./h)	12.7 ± 12.2	3.5 - 58.3	9.4 ± 6.6	0.3 - 29.4	0.0161

Significant differences (paired t-test, $p<0.01$) between pretreatment and posttreatment values are underlined.

Table 6. Comparison of sleep data with and without the appliance among supine, lateral and prone groups

	Supine Group (n=44)			Lateral Group (n=15)			Prone Group (n=13)		
	Without	With	P value	Without	With	P value	Without	With	P value
Respiratory function variables									
Apnea-hypopnea index (No./h)	47.8 ± 26.1	14.3 ± 12.2	<u>0.0001</u>	56.4 ± 12.7	45.0 ± 13.3	0.0538	<u>16.1 ± 11.5</u>	<u>9.9 ± 4.8</u>	<u>0.0029</u>
Apnea index (No./h)	28.3 ± 17.0	6.5 ± 7.3	<u>0.0001</u>	37.7 ± 22.9	27.9 ± 13.4	0.0593	6.2 ± 5.5	<u>2.0 ± 1.5</u>	<u>0.0011</u>
Mean event duration (s)	23.9 ± 5.8	22.0 ± 4.4	<u>0.0133</u>	23.7 ± 5.2	23.4 ± 5.5	0.4823	21.1 ± 5.3	17.9 ± 3.3	0.0205
Longest event duration (s)	<u>80.9 ± 39.1</u>	<u>69.1 ± 22.9</u>	<u>0.0012</u>	88.9 ± 42.9	73.1 ± 13.9	0.1727	57.9 ± 20.0	30.7 ± 8.0	0.0170
Mean oxgen saturation (%)	92.0 ± 2.6	93.1 ± 1.8	<u>0.0014</u>	91.0 ± 3.6	92.3 ± 2.5	0.0455	93.9 ± 0.53	94.6 ± 1.0	0.0395
Minimal oxygen saturation (%)	71.5 ± 12.9	75.2 ± 9.7	0.0334	68.4 ± 6.5	72.4 ± 8.3	0.0403	78.5 ± 0.85	78.8 ± 2.6	0.5244
Sleep quality variables									
Total sleep time (min)	444.0 ± 94.7	452.8 ± 88.2	0.0909	421.6 ± 98.6	443.4 ± 19.2	0.8969	420.1 ± 130.7	484.8 ± 46.2	0.0849
Supine sleep (%)	70.0 ± 36.8	70.3 ± 30.2	0.3788	49.9 ± 25.6	32.0 ± 38.1	0.3860	13.2 ± 11.6	6.0 ± 10.8	0.7428
Lateral sleep (%)	15.5 ± 14.3	26.5 ± 28.4	0.0879	39.8 ± 18.2	34.7 ± 39.2	0.6248	11.1 ± 9.2	14.0 ± 25.7	0.5613
Prone sleep (%)	14.5 ± 34.2	3.2 ± 4.8	0.3208	10.5 ± 13.8	30.7 ± 42.6	0.2418	75.7 ± 19.8	80.0 ± 36.8	0.7865
Stage 1 sleep (%)	14.7 ± 5.4	<u>12.1 ± 7.5</u>	<u>0.0012</u>	27.6 ± 19.5	19.3 ± 9.1	0.0748	<u>23.9 ± 4.5</u>	<u>13.8 ± 1.2</u>	<u>0.0001</u>
Stage 2 sleep (%)	47.4 ± 15.5	48.0 ± 16.1	0.0533	36.0 ± 8.1	38.6 ± 15.6	0.5755	51.9 ± 8.9	47.7 ± 11.0	0.1615
Stage 3 sleep (%)	8.2 ± 10.3	5.9 ± 2.9	0.4997	4.2 ± 3.4	5.7 ± 0.22	0.1424	5.4 ± 4.1	8.0 ± 3.7	0.1738
Stage 4 sleep (%)	5.5 ± 8.6	4.7 ± 7.4	0.0606	0.82 ± 0.71	2.6 ± 3.0	0.1080	<u>1.6 ± 2.6</u>	<u>2.5 ± 3.5</u>	<u>0.0078</u>
Rapid eye movement sleep (%)	9.3 ± 7.8	<u>17.0 ± 5.5</u>	<u>0.0001</u>	15.2 ± 9.4	10.1 ± 3.6	0.0570	<u>3.8 ± 5.0</u>	<u>14.1 ± 2.4</u>	<u>0.0001</u>
Arousal index (No./h)	15.3 ± 15.2	<u>10.5 ± 8.8</u>	<u>0.0055</u>	11.3 ± 1.8	9.0 ± 3.5	0.2942	<u>6.5 ± 2.4</u>	<u>5.0 ± 2.1</u>	<u>0.0009</u>

Significant differences (paired t-test, p<0.01) between pretreatment and posttreatment values are underlined.

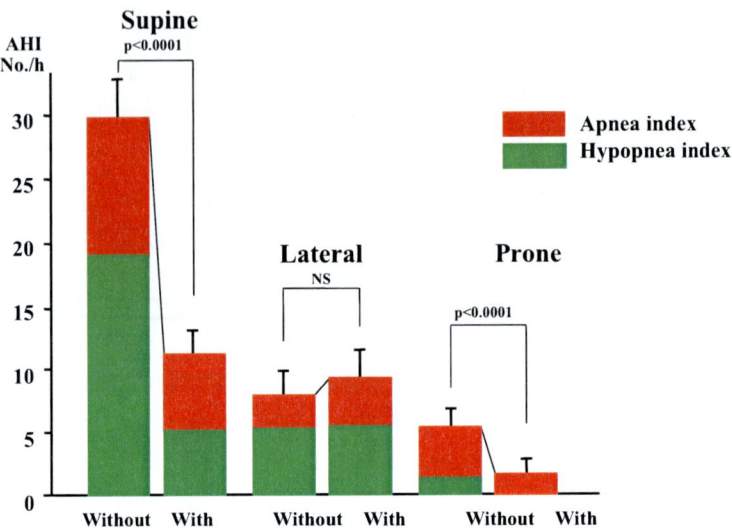

Figure 16. Comparison of mean apnea-hypopnea index (AHI) change in each sleep posture with and without oral appliance. AHI in the supine and prone positions was also significantly reduced, while in the lateral position it was increased slightly. Error bars=standard error.

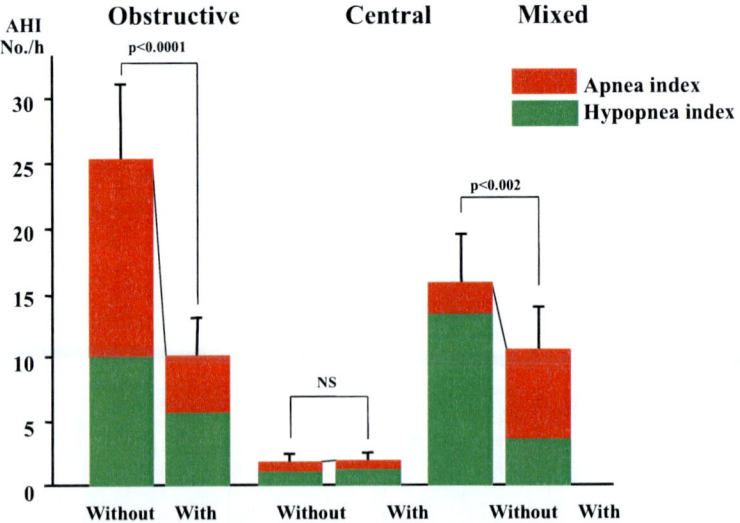

Figure 17. Mean obstructive, central, and mixed AHI changes with and without oral appliance. Obstructive and mixed AHI was significantly reduced. Central AHI was increased, but not significantly. Error bars=standard error.

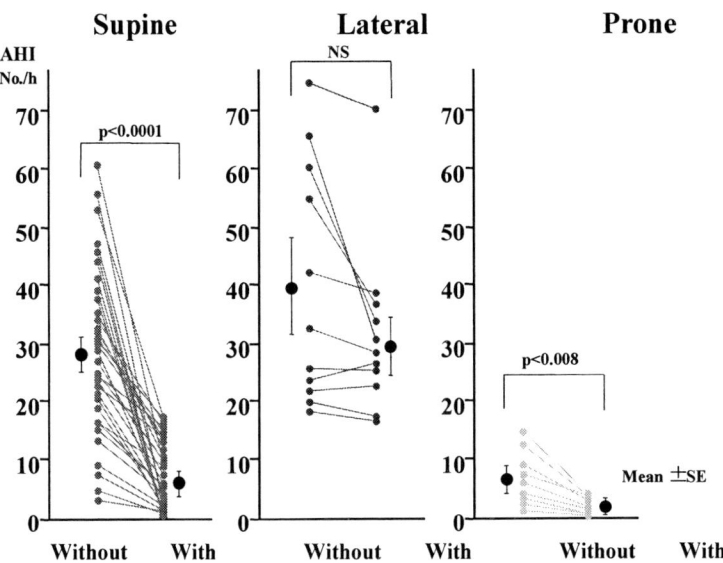

Figure 18. Comparison of mean AHI Change with and without device of each patient in supine, lateral and prone groups. Pretreatment mean AHI of lateral group (n=15) was significantly (ANOVA) higher than those of supine (n=44) and prone (n=13) groups. All groups showed reduction of mean AHI. Differences were significant (paired t-test) in the supine and prone groups, and not significant in the lateral group. Error bars=standard deviation.

Forty-four (61.1 %, 7 women and 37 men) of the 72 patients exhibited apneas most frequently in the supine position, 15 patients (20.8 %, 1 woman and 14 men) in the lateral decubitus position, and 13 patients (18.1 %, 2 women and 11 men) in the prone position. The patients in the supine group were significantly (p<0.0001, ANOVA) younger (48.5 ± 4.0 years, range 37-54 years) than those in the lateral group (63.6 ± 10.6 years, range 48-72 years) and the prone group (p<0.0002, 57.6 ± 8.8 years, range 47-72 years). The body mass index (28.2 ± 3.0, 29.2 ± 3.5, and 26.5 ± 2.7 kg/m^2) was not significantly different.

The mean polysomnographic values with and without the appliance in each group are listed in Table 6. AHI was significantly lower in the prone group than in the lateral group (p<0.0001, ANOVA) or the supine group (p<0.002). In the supine group the total AHI (Figure 18) decreased significantly. Treatment was successful (AHI<10) in 27 of the 44 patients (61.4 %). Thirty-seven patients (84.1 %) showed a 50 % reduction of AHI.

In the lateral group (Figure 18), total AHI was reduced, but not significantly. No patients attained the normal range (AHI<10) even after insertion of the appliance. One (6.7 %) of the 15 patients showed a 50 % reduction of AHI.

In the prone group (Figure 18) AHI was reduced significantly by the device. Treatment was successful (AHI<10) in 11 (84.6 %) of the 13 patients. Six patients (46.2 %) showed a 50 % reduction of AHI.

Total sleep time revealed no significant difference among the three groups (Table 6).

The longest sleep position was supine in the supine and lateral groups and prone in the prone group (Table 6). The proportion of each position in each group did not differ significantly even after use of the device. In the supine group, sleep efficiency was improved significantly and stage 1 sleep was reduced significantly. In the prone group, stage 1 sleep was reduced significantly, and stage 4 sleep was increased significantly (Table 6). Rapid eye movement sleep was increased significantly in the supine and prone groups. Arousal index was decreased significantly in the supine and prone groups (Table 6).

The present study placed emphasis on the relationship between sleep position and occurrence of apneic or hypopneic episodes, although the criteria for clinical treatment success should include parameters relating to improvement in oxygenation, sleep architecture, day time sleepiness and snoring along with the respiratory parameters. In this study two criteria, a fall in AHI to < 10 and a 50 % reduction in AHI, were used, as AHI differed significantly among the groups. A cutoff point based on the AHI in percent may underestimate the efficacy in mild cases and overestimate it in severe cases. In contrast, the reduction in the AHI to < 10 shows a reverse tendency because patients with severe apneas will find it more difficult to reach the range than those with mild apnea.

The genioglossal muscle [59, 89, 98, 99], the masseter muscle, and the inferior head of the lateral pterygoid muscle [59, 89, 99] showed significantly lower electromyographic amplitudes during and higher amplitudes after obstructive apnea. Hypotonia of the muscles and the weight of the mandible, particularly in the supine position, can lead to opening of the mouth and further dorsal displacement of the mandible and tongue, resulting in pharyngeal narrowing and increased airway resistance, and finally obstructive apnea [59, 89, 99]. The positional apnea patients, whose AHI is twice higher in the supine than in the lateral posture, were found to differ from unselected apneic patients in a larger posterior airway space, less elongated soft palate and somewhat more prominent retrognathia [100]. It is known that CPAP pressure levels often need to be higher with the patients in the supine position compared to all other positions.

During the CPAP titration procedure patients are specifically asked to sleep in the supine position to insure that CPAP will be effective in all sleep positions. Effectiveness of the oral appliance therapy must take into account the same factors as CPAP therapy.

Gravity on the mandible, tongue and other tissues which attach to the mandible seems to play a minor role in the prone position. In the prone position, the pressure by a pillow or mattress on the mandible might lead to passive mandibular retrusion and further dorsal displacement of the base of the tongue. The prone sleep position was associated with an increased risk of sudden infant death syndrome [101] as a result of oropharyngeal obstruction [102] and obstructive apnea secondary to partial nasal obstruction [103]. The inferior head of the lateral pterygoid muscle protruding the mandible showed significantly lower electromyographic activity during obstructive apnea than before it [59, 89]. The relaxation of the prime protruder of the mandible could result in mandibular retrusion by dorsal pressure on it.

The effects of gravity and passive pressure on the mandible in the lateral position seem to be smaller than in the other positions. Patients who show apneic events chiefly in the lateral position are apt to be obese and severe. For such patients, it is unlikely that the oral appliance will be effective. Other therapies such as CPAP or surgery combined with weight loss might be more appropriate.

Oral appliances appear to be less effective when the respiratory disturbance index exceeds 40 to 50 per hour, or AHI of > 60 [65]. A recent study reported that the success rate of oral appliance therapy correlated inversely to disease severity [20]. However, in the present study efficiency and disease severity showed no significant correlation. This inconsistency can be explained by the fact that most of the patients in the present study had markedly more severe apneas than those in the other studies. One possibility for the poor beneficial effect in the severe cases is the site of obstruction. Wide areas of obstruction extending from the soft palate or uvula to the base of the tongue or epiglottis [104] are seen more frequently in severe apnea patients than in mild cases. The length of the soft palate correlated inversely to the success rate of oral appliance therapy [19]. Large obstructions below the uvular level could not be eliminated by the device. The other possibility for the low success rate in severe apnea cases is sleep posture. Marked obesity proved to be related to fluctuating results from night to night in AHI in the lateral position [105]. Kavey et al. [106] pointed out that the reports of inconsistent success of treatments are attributable in part to hidden factors such as sleep position. The inter- and intra-individual differences of efficiency of the oral appliance, particularly in severe and obese cases, could be related to the fact that the results are strongly influenced by sleep posture. Sleep position recording by polysomnography is important not only for the selection of treatment method, but also for prediction of posttreatment evaluation of effectiveness of oral appliance therapy. Very obese apnea patients showed high AHI even on the sides, so favoring the lateral position may not be as beneficial as previously thought [107]. Without attention to the apnea index in the supine, lateral and prone sleep postures one could easily mistakenly assess treatment as effective or ineffective based on the changes in the apnea index resulting solely from a change in sleep position [106].

a.5. Prognosis

If the patient had muscle or temporomandibular joint discomfort just after the first use of the appliance, the adverse effects resolved within several days to several weeks with regular use. If the symptoms continued longer, the appliance was separated and rejoined at a decreased protrusive position. The adjustment was repeated until all discomforts disappeared. Polysomnographic recording with the appliance was performed after the habituation period.

Treatment adherence is variable, with patients reporting using the appliance a median of 77 % of nights at 1 year [31]. 46 % of patients were objectively using CPAP for a mean of 106.9 days at least 4 hours per night on 70 % of the nights [24]. 30 months after CPAP prescription, only 50 % of patients accepted CPAP [108]. Our previous longitudinal study revealed that a similar appliance maintained its efficacy in all patients without significant temporomandibular joint problems with a mean length of follow-up of 55 months (range 24 to 96 months) [109]. Compliance in a previous study was approximately 90 %, followed for 2.5 years [22]. The disadvantage of the rigid type appliance is that the splints must be repositioned after separation if the patient shows insufficient results or temporomandibular joint symptoms. However this study revealed higher longitudinal compliance than that of the Herbst appliance (52 % after 3 years) [18]. The non-adjustable appliance (Figure 5a,b,c) has higher compliance than an adjustable appliance (Figure 6c). Compliance was about 90 % followed for 5 years and higher in comparison to CPAP. In more than half of patients the oral appliance showed sufficient effectiveness and they used only the oral appliance [9]. Some patients used CPAP daily and the oral appliance during business trips or travel. Some other patients simultaneously used CPAP and oral appliance (Figure 12). It may be prudent for the dentist to evaluate each patient every 6 months for the first several years. Further careful follow-up data are necessary to define the long-term efficacy, the risk of complications and the need for adjustment of the appliance.

b. Maxillofacial Surgical Treatment

Surgery is generally indicated when applicable conservative therapies are unsuccessful or not tolerated, as well as for patients who have an identifiable underlying surgically correctable abnormality that is causing the SAS [110]. The three major anatomic regions of potential collapse during sleep in SAS patients are the nose, palate, and tongue base. Examination of the oral cavity should include an evaluation of dental health, class of occlusion, and the characteristics of the oral mucous membranes and tongue. The pharynx should be examined by assessing the length of the soft palate, any lateral pharyngeal redundancy, and the size of the tonsils. Cephalometric radiographs assist in the overall evaluation of the soft tissue and bony configuration. However, such cephalometric evaluation is limited because the patient is evaluated while awake and seated, and because it is not a dynamic study obtained during sleep. Surgical procedures that are considered include uvulopalatopharyngoplasty, laser midline glossectomy and lingualplasty, inferior sagittal mandibular osteotomy and genioglossal advancement with hyoid myotomy and suspension, maxillomandibular osteotomy and advancement, and tracheotomy.

An epidermoid or dermatoid cyst in the sublingual area can press the tongue posteriorly and result in apnea and snoring (Figure 19a, b). An extremely large mandibular torus can also cause apnea (Figure 19c, d). Symptoms will improve if the mandibular torus or cyst are removed. Tongue reduction surgery can be performed in SAS patients with macroglossia. If a SAS patient is not obese, and there is no obvious problem in the otolaryngeal region, an abnormality may be recognized in the stomatognathic system, and the diagnosis of the oral surgeon is important.

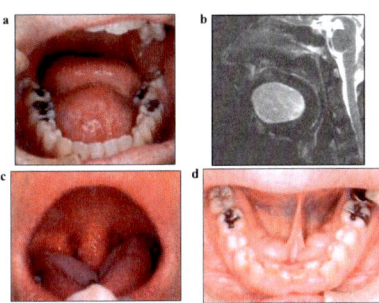

Figure 19. Structural problems in the oral cavity resulting in SAS. Epidermoid or dermoid cyst (a,b) in sublingual region, excessive large uvula (c) and mandibular torus (d) can cause SAS.

b.1. Orthognathic Surgery

Here, the author focuses on the stomatognathic region. The Powell-Riley surgical protocol is a two-phase procedure that directs surgical treatment toward the specific regions of obstruction during sleep [111]. Phase I of the surgical intervention includes nasal reconstruction, uvulopalatopharyngoplasty, and a limited mandibular osteotomy with genioglossus advancement-hyoid myotomy and suspension. Phase II represents skeletal reconstruction and consists of bi-maxillary advancement, commonly referred to as maxillary and mandibular osteotomy. Surgery for SAS is primarily aimed at enlarging the airway while decreasing its collapsibility. Several different protocols for surgical treatment in SAS have been adopted. Prinsell [112] adopted a "site-specific" approach in which patients with "orohypopharyngeal narrowing caused by macroglossia with a retropositioned tongue base" are considered eligible for maxillomandibular advancement surgery. Mandibular advancement surgery such as sagittal splitting osteotomy, which is a representative orthognathic surgical method, can be used to treat SAS of congenital micrognathia like Pierre Robin's sequence (Figure 20) [113], Treacher Collins syndrome and Hallermann-Streiff syndrome (Figure 21).

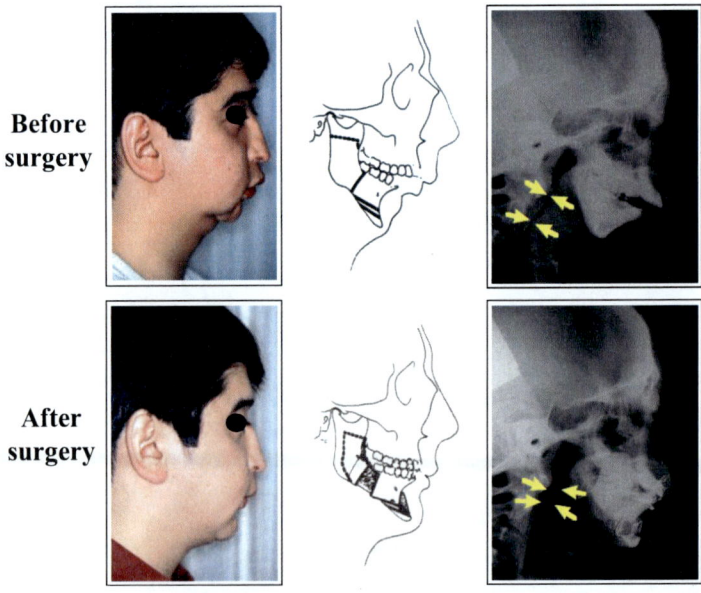

Figure 20. A patient with sleep-disordered breathing due to micrognathia related to Pierre Robin Complex. His mandible was advanced by performing sagittal splitting osteotomy and genioplasty and the respiratory symptom and esthetic problem were improved [113].

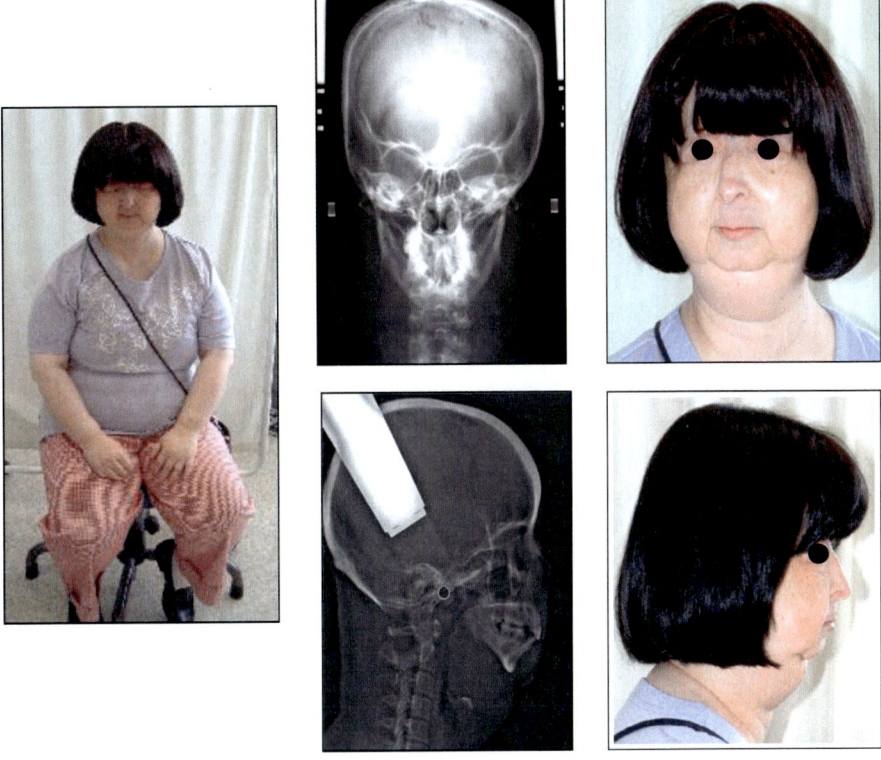

Figure 21. A patient with Hallermann-Streiff syndrome with sleep-disordered breathing. The patient has an extremely small mandible and showed severe SAS with AHI of 70-90.

Maxillomandibular advancement surgery for SAS patients consists of a bilateral sagittal splitting osteotomy of the mandible and a Le Fort I osteotomy of the maxilla. Maxillomandibular advancement surgery is regarded as the most effective and acceptable surgical procedure for SAS with a success rate of 75 % to 100 % [37, 114-116]. However, the results are based on varying criteria such as a postoperative AHI of less than 20 or a greater than 50 % reduction in AHI [37], less than 15 [117], less than 10 [114], less than 15 or a reduction in AHI and AI of greater than 60 % [37]. The current technique of sagittal splitting ramus osteotomy follows descriptions published by Obwegeser in 1964 [118]. Today, sagittal splitting ramus osteotomy is the most commonly used procedure in the treatment of maxillofacial deformities such as prognathism or retrognathism. Le Fort I maxillary osteotomy is a common orthognathic surgical procedure. A transverse separation of the dentoalveolar process of the maxilla to include the palate, floor of the nose, and the maxillary sinuses in order to widen, narrow, lengthen, shorten, or level the upper jaw is done so that it can be placed in harmony with the other facial bones, as well as the skull.

b.2. Distraction Osteogenesis

Distraction osteogenesis is a technique in which bone can be lengthened by de novo bone formation as part of the normal healing process that occurs between surgically osteomized bone segments. Distraction osteogenesis is playing a rapidly expanding role in the treatment of airway obstruction and craniofacial deformities resulting from mandibular deficiency. Mandibular distraction osteogenesis is frequently performed in apneic children [119, 120] with congenital anomalies, and also in adults [121]. Compared with orthognathic surgery, distraction osteogenesis has advantages such as less surgical stress and invasion, no need for bone grafting, induction of soft tissue adaptation, and more extensive bone lengthening. However, it requires more time for the lengthening and formation of the bone. We are now able to extend across difficult long distances, which is impossible with mandibular advancement surgery, by applying distraction osteogenesis (Figure 22) [122].

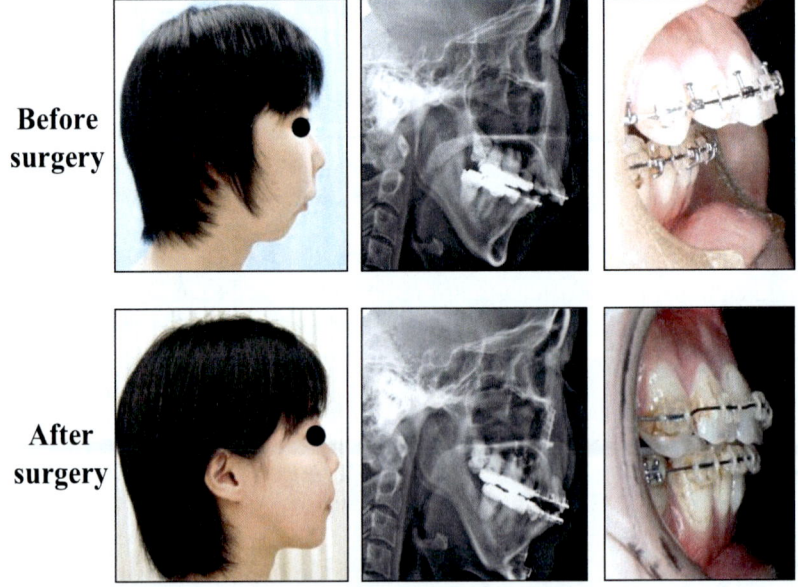

Figure 22. Mandible was advanced in a patient with micrognathia 0.8mm per day and totally 14mm in 18 days after corticotomy of the mandible [122].

3. FUTURE DIRECTIONS

a. Periodontal Disease and SAS

Periodontal diseases are very prevalent and affect 50-90% of the global population. Periodontitis is a chronic infection by oral bacteria that affects the supporting structures of the teeth and is a major cause of tooth loss in adults [123]. A mechanism has been proposed whereby the burden of bacterial pathogens, antigens, endotoxins, and inflammatory cytokines in periodontitis contributes to the process of atherogenesis and thromboembolic events. In response to infection and inflammation, susceptible individuals may exhibit greater expression of local and systemic mediators and may thereby be at increased risk for a myocardial infarction or stroke [124].

a.1. SAS as a Risk Factor for Periodontal Disease

Periodontal diseases are caused by microorganisms such as *Porphyromonas gingivalis*, *Actinobacillus actinomycetemcomitans*, and *Treponema denticola* that colonize the tooth surface at or below the gingival margin. In a patient with 28 teeth with pocket depths of 6-7 mm and bone loss, the subgingival surface area of infection could be roughly similar to the surface area represented by both hands [123]. The subgingival bacteria in deep periodontal pockets exist in a highly organized biofilm. Subgingival biofilms represent a large and continuing bacterial load and are a constant source of lipopolysaccharides, as well as Gram-negative bacteria, to the blood stream. Proinflammatory cytokines can reach high concentrations in the tissues of the periodontium. A mechanism has been proposed whereby the burden of bacterial pathogens, antigens, endotoxins, and inflammatory cytokines in periodontitis contributes to the process of atherogenesis and thromboembolic events. In response to infection and inflammation, susceptible individuals may exhibit greater expression of local and systemic mediators and may thereby be at increased risk for a myocardial infarction or stroke [123].

It has become clear that the majority of SAS patients have periodontal disease (Table 7). In a study by the author [124], the average number of remaining teeth was 26.2. The number of teeth observed to be bleeding by probing showed an average of 5.9. The ratio of moderate periodontal disease having pockets of 4-6mm was 38.4%, and 58.9% showed severe periodontal disease presenting 6mm at the deepest pocket. Patients with periodontal pockets equal to or less than 3mm accounted for only 2.7% of the patients receiving periodical periodontal treatment. The results are based on patients mainly with slight to moderate SAS.

Most patients are referred to an expert in sleep medical care who understands that manufacture of an oral appliance is difficult with few teeth. Most patients have periodontal disease with medium or severe grade symptoms, who have not received periodical periodontal treatment. It seems that the ratio of severe periodontal disease increases when we include severe CPAP-managed SAS patients. The reasons why periodontal disease is observed at a high frequency in many SAS patients are the prevalence of both diseases after middle-age, obesity, diabetes mellitus, dryness of the oral cavity due to snoring, diet problems, and excessive occlusal force because of bruxism related to sleep apnea (Figure 23).

Table 7. Ratio of periodontal disease and lifestyle-related diseases in 219 SAS patients.

SAS patients	Mean ± SD
Mean age (years)	53.4 ± 13.8
Patients (female:male)	219 (156:63)
Mean AHI (No./h)	19.1 ± 16.5
Periodontal status	
Mean pocket depth less than 3mm (%)	2.7
Mean pocket depth 4 -6mm (%)	58.9
Mean pocket depth over 6mm (%)	38.4
Remaining teeth (No.)	26.2 ± 3.8
Bleeding by probing (No.)	6.5 ± 8.3
Other lifestyle-related diseases	
Obesity (%)	52.1
Hypertension (%)	39.7
Diabetes mellitus (%)	20.5
Heart disease (%)	20.5
Hyperlipidemia (%)	19.2

The ratio of moderate periodontal disease having pockets 4-6mm was 38.4%, and 58.9% of severe periodontal disease patients presenting pockets deeper than 6mm. Patients having periodontal pockets equal to or less than 3mm were only 2.7%, and all had had periodical periodontal treatment. All patients who had not received periodical periodontal treatment had periodontal disease and morbidity was higher than the rates for lifestyle-related diseases such as hypertension or diabetes mellitus

SAS may be a risk factor for periodontal disease [124]. The relationship among periodontal disease and obesity [125], diabetes mellitus [126] and coronary heart disease has been elucidated. SAS could become an exacerbation factor for a lifestyle-related disease, and obesity is an important risk factor for SAS [124]. If one becomes obese and the internal organs accumulate fat, it increases the risk of developing diabetes mellitus, hyperlipidemia, high blood pressure, and arteriosclerosis. Furthermore, developing coronary heart disease that aggregates these conditions is called metabolic syndrome, and a relationship between SAS and metabolic syndrome has gradually been clarified.

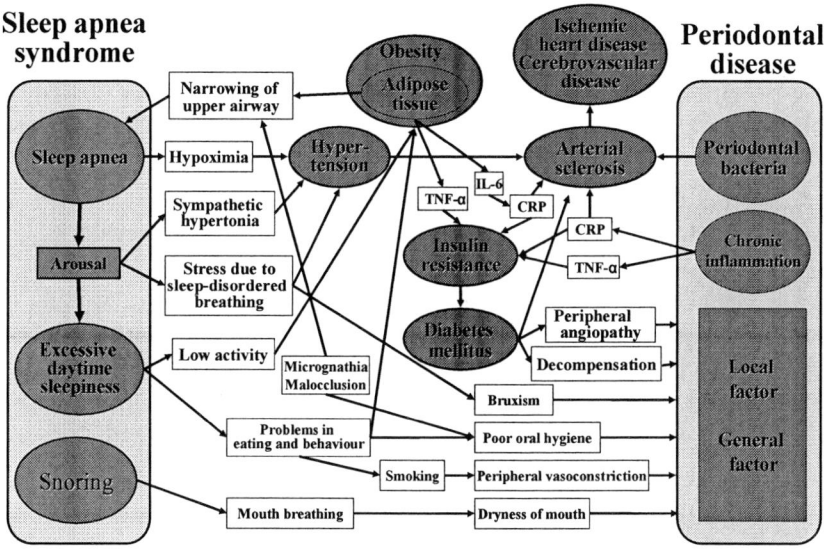

Figure 23. Relationship between periodontal disease and sleep apnea syndrome. SAS acts as an aggravating risk factor of periodontal disease. Periodontal disease or SAS as life-related disease can aggravate a series of life-related diseases.

Periodontal disease exacerbates lifestyle-related diseases due to slight chronic inflammation, and can aggravate these diseases (Figure 23). In other words, metabolism disorders due to diabetes mellitus and peripheral angiopathy exacerbate periodontal disease. In addition, air is taken in directly via the mouth, and mouth respiration with snoring causes a drying of the gingiva and oral mucosa. This seems to promote progression of periodontal disease so that the self-cleansing and gingival tissue resistance fails. It is thought that "canned coffee syndrome", or drinking large quantities of canned coffee with too much sugar to avoid excessive daytime sleepiness in SAS patients has a bad influence on diabetes mellitus, obesity and periodontal disease. Powerful forces act on teeth in bruxism related to sleep stress and these also accelerate periodontal tissue destruction (Figure 23).

a.2. Relationship among Periodontal Disease, Diabetes Mellitus and Heart Disease

Diabetes mellitus is a common, multifactorial disease process involving genetic, environmental and behavioral risk factors. The chronic condition is marked by defects in glucose metabolism that produce hyperglycemia in patients. The number of Japanese patients with type 2 diabetes (non-insulin-dependent diabetes mellitus) is markedly increasing. This may be due to the rapid Westernization of the lifestyle in Japan. Obesity is the greatest risk factor for diabetes mellitus. Fat cells (adipocytes) in obese patients secrete many cytokines such as tumor necrosis factor (TNF- α), interleukin-6 (IL-6) and leptin. TNF- α is also produced by monocytes or macrophages and plays an important role in inflammation reactions, and it is known to induce insulin resistance [127]. TNF- α is produced by periodontal pockets with chronic periodontal inflammation. It is reported that the serum TNF- α of diabetics is reduced by successful periodontal treatment, and subsequently insulin resistance was improved. It is thought that obesity and diabetes mellitus are important risk factors for periodontal disease. Also, a significant correlation between obesity and periodontal disease is reported [125]. Periodontal disease can induce insulin resistance, and, after initiation, act as promoting factor. It is possible that periodontal disease developing as complication of obesity or diabetes mellitus becomes an aggravating factor for diabetes due to chronic inflammation. The increase in type 2 diabetes mellitus in Asia differs from that reported in other parts of the world: it has developed in a much shorter time, in a younger age group, and in people with much lower body-mass index. There are not so many markedly obese patients with diabetes mellitus in Japan compared with Westerners. This suggests that periodontal disease might exacerbate diabetes mellitus in Japan.

Transient bacteremia can occur due to not only surgical procedures such as extraction of a tooth, but also conservative procedures such as tartar removal. When periodontal bacteria stick to the endocardium and proliferate, it can result in infective endocarditis. The most frequently detected bacteria in infective endocarditis is oral streptococus. Periodontal bacteria are also detected in the tissue of arteriosclerosis.

Coronary heart disease is the most frequent cause of death in diabetics. It has become clear that chronic inflammation participates in the initiation of arteriosclerosis and coronary heart disease, and that C- reactive protein (CRP) promotes aggravation of vascular lesions [128]. CRP acts on the vascular endothelium, and is a promotion factor in arteriosclerosis. The CRP level increases when people are infected by periodontal bacteria. In addition, interleukin-6 of adipose tissue origin induces CRP production from hepatocytes.

Severe periodontal disease may thus have an influence on the development of arteriosclerosis (Figure 23).

a.3. Relationship between Periodontal Disease and Metabolic Syndrome

Lifestyle-related diseases are defined as diseases that appear to increase in frequency as countries become more industrialized and people live longer. They include Alzheimer's disease, atherosclerosis, cancer, chronic liver disease or cirrhosis, chronic obstructive pulmonary disease, type 2 diabetes, heart disease, nephritis or chronic renal failure, osteoporosis, stroke, and obesity. "Healthy Japan 21" targeted the primary prevention of lifestyle-related disease, and it was devised in 2000 by the Minister of Health, Labour and Welfare of Japan. Nine fields including nourishment and eating habits, physical activity and exercise, rest and mental health, smoking, alcohol, dental health, diabetes mellitus, cardiovascular disease, and cancer were chosen. Periodontal disease was chosen along with obesity, hypertension and diabetes mellitus and came to be recognized as a lifestyle-related disease. Most SAS patients suffer from diabetes mellitus, obesity, hypertension, hyperlipidemia, and cardiovascular disease. SAS can become an exacerbating factor for other lifestyle-related diseases. Japanese suffer from SAS more easily compared with Westerners due to their craniofacial morphology characteristics, even if they are not so obese, but about 70% of Japanese SAS patients are also obese. Obesity is an important risk factor for SAS. In addition, SAS is considered to be one of the factors for hypertension. Metabolic syndrome is a combination of medical disorders that increases the risk of cardiovascular disease and diabetes [129]. It affects a large number of people in a clustered fashion. In some studies, the prevalence in the USA is calculated as being up to 25% of the population. The relationship between SAS and metabolic syndrome has gradually been clarified. Periodontal disease is observed in almost all patients as a complication of an SAS lifestyle-related disease, and it occurs at the highest frequency (Table 7). Periodontal disease promotes lifestyle-related disease via slight chronic inflammation, and can augment disease progression even if the degree of obesity is low (Figure 23) [124].

a.4. Oral appliance Therapy of SAS and Oral Hygiene

When a patient is referred for oral appliance therapy for SAS, dentists should be aware that periodontal disease is a lifestyle-related disease and that it promotes other diseases. It is necessary to treat periodontal disease [124]. It is important not to disturb self-purification of saliva when we make an oral appliance and not to cover the gingival margin with any device. In addition, it is important to design oral appliances that reduce discomfort and minimize bruxism. It is also important to restrain mouth breathing, and not to dry the oral cavity. We should follow-up periodontal disease along with a periodical follow-up of oral appliances. A patient unaware of SAS and lifestyle-related disease can have a checkup at a dentist for dental treatment (Figure 24).

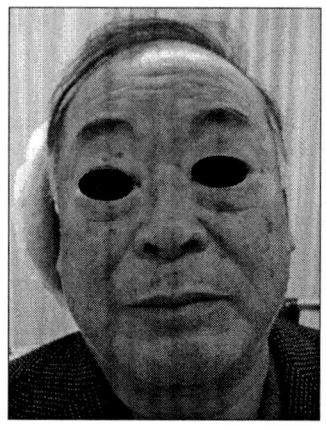
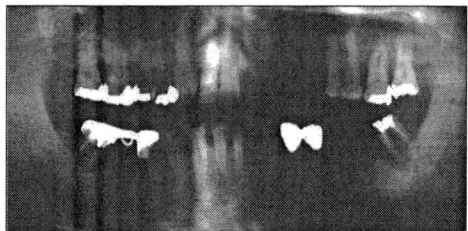

Figure 24. A seventy-year old man was referred to our hospital with chief complaint of discomfort in the oral cavity at the time of getting up. His oral hygiene was extremely bad, absorption of alveolar bone was observed, and he was diagnosed as a severe periodontal disease. There were obesity, snoring, daytime sleepiness, too, and SAS was suspected. As a result of sleep study, he was diagnosed as moderate SAS. As a result of blood examination, diabetes mellitus, hyperlipemia became clear, too. It is important for us to cooperate and perform dental treatment and treatment of internal medicine for lifestyle-related diseases such as diabetes mellitus for such cases.

It is necessary for dentists to refer SAS patients with other lifestyle-related diseases for diagnosis and treatment. In addition, dentists should recognize that the majority of SAS patients have periodontal disease and that it can worsen a series of lifestyle-related diseases. It seems meaningful to recommend appropriate dental treatment for patients using CPAP in departments of respiratory medicine or otolaryngology. Recently, the influence of periodontal disease on these diseases and the role of periodontal treatment have been clarified [123]. It is now clear that blood pressure falls significantly after oral appliance treatment [66]. However, the influence on lifestyle-related diseases of periodontal disease in SAS patients, and the changes in condition of patients after oral appliance treatment have not been clarified.

This will become a significant clinical issue in the future and medical departments and dentistry departments must cooperate to elucidate the relevance of these diseases [124].

b. Central Mechanism of SAS and the Effect of Oral Appliances

It is necessary to consider the cortical control activity over the stomatognathic system and have a perception of the oropharynx region when considering the occurrence of sleep apnea. The author measured movement-related cortical potential and contingent negative variation to examine cortical control with jaw movement [130, 131].

Contingent negative variation accompanying a jaw and tongue protrusion task, was measured revealing a difference in the amplitude and distribution of response in SAS patients [9, 124]. Magnetoencephalography has a very high time and space resolving power. The author used a magnetometer to assess the soft palate and record a somatosensory magnetic field, and observed the reaction in second somatosensory field on both sides [132], as well as the reaction reduction during sleep [9, 124]. In addition, the authors measured the brain blood volume with near-infrared spectroscopy, jaw closing and opening movements, tongue protrusion movement, a measurement at the time of pronunciation, brain blood volume changes during sleep, and those in the frontal lobe during a word fluency task [124].

In the future, such non-invasive brain function measurements will provide new information on the central mechanism of SAS occurrence, its changes related to oral appliance therapy, and choice of oral appliance therapy.

c. Future Oral Appliance

The author has treated over 2,000 patients with SAS using mainly oral appliances [9, 19, 22, 39]. The patients sometimes experienced a transitory discomfort of the masticatory muscle or temporomandibular joint, excessive salivation, and transient tooth discomfort after first using the device. It would be very meaningful to develop a new treatment device with fewer complications for safe and long-term use. The author aims to develop a device which allows free jaw movements during sleep and advance the mandible if sleep apnea occurs based on respiratory pattern sensing. The device could be combined with CPAP. When sleep apnea occurs, the device protrudes the mandible, and even if the apnea disappears, the positive airway pressure additionally works to diminish any remaining upper airway obstruction. The device could minimize the airway pressure because it prevents patients from mouth breathing, air-leak, and upper airway collapse by advancing the lower jaw. Many patients with severe SAS have been intolerant to CPAP because of discomfort related to the high pressure sensation and air-leak. This device will be highly beneficial for such patients and patients with poor compliance with standard CPAP or other oral appliances [124].

Chapter 2

NEUROPHYSIOLOGICAL ASPECT OF SLEEP APNEA SYNDROME

The stomatognathtic system is involved in various functions such as chewing, swallowing, digestion, respiration and speech. Little is known about the direct effect of oral function on the central nervous system, possibly because brain-imaging methods have difficulty in obtaining satisfactory images influenced by head motion related jaw movement. The cortical mechanism mediating even simple mandibular movements still remains uncertain. It has become clear from studies of the effect of ablation [133], electrical stimulation and single neuron recordings [134, 135] in monkeys that two cortical areas, the primary face motor area and the cortical masticatory area, are involved in jaw movement, but their mechanisms in humans have not been explored precisely. Electromyograms (surface or intramuscular) have been used to study jaw and upper airway muscles during sleep. Electroencephalograms (movement-related cortical potentials or contingent negative variation) were used in an attempt to elucidate the role of the cerebral cortex in the control of movements and the cognitive process in preparation for a response directed to a purpose.

1. ELECTROPHYSIOLOGICAL STUDIES

a. Electromyogram

To evaluate the efficiency of the oral appliance, the activity of masticatory and tongue muscles was investigated polysomnographically with and without the appliance. Fifteen patients (3 women and 12 men) with SAS, between the ages of

45 and 72 years (mean age 54.0 ± 8.4 years) were evaluated polysomnographically [59].

Surface Ag/AgCl electrodes (EP12, Unique Medical, Tokyo, Japan) for the genioglossal muscle were placed midsagittally, midway between the mental protuberance and lower lip, and midway between the inner aspect of the mandible and hyoid bone (Figure 25) [59, 89]. Ag/AgCl electrodes were also used over the masseter muscle 15 mm apart in the direction of the main fibers. Two polyurethane coated fine wire electrodes (0.08 mm in diameter, Unique Medical, Japan) within a 60 mm long 23-gauge injection needle (0.65 mm in diameter, Terumo, Japan) were used through an intraoral route to record EMG activity from the inferior head of the lateral pterygoid muscle (Figure 26) [89]. The tips of these fine wire electrodes were exposed 1 mm and bent 3 mm and 5 mm into a hook from the tip. The wire electrodes were attached to the buccal face of the maxillary premolar with adhesive wax led out of the corner of the mouth to avoid movement artifacts [89]. The EMG signals were amplified with a band pass of 30 to 3000 Hz and with a 200 ms time constant. Polysomnographic recordings were performed.

During obstructive sleep apnea, airflow disappeared, but abdominal and chest movements remained partially (Figure 27). The genioglossal, masseter and lateral pterygoid muscles showed apparently reduced activity during obstructive sleep apnea (Figure 27).

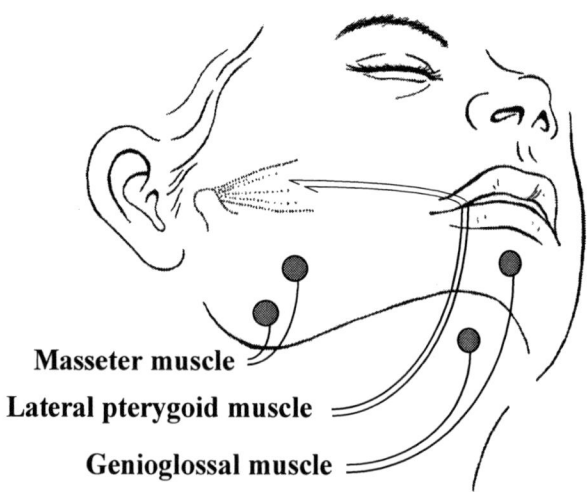

Figure 25. Electrode placement for the masseter, lateral pterygoid and genioglossal muscles. Surface electrodes were used for the genioglossal and masseter muscles. Fine wire electrodes were applied for the lateral pterygoid muscle.

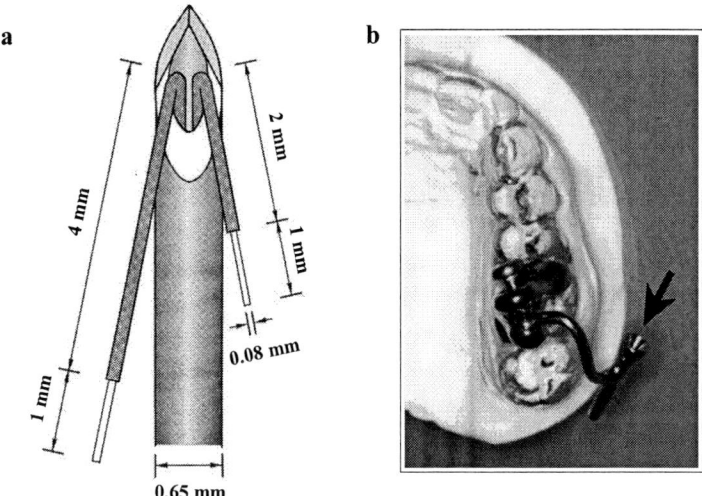

Figure 26. Fine wire electrodes in the needle (a) and intraoral appliance for lateral pterygoid muscle EMG recording (b). Two polyurethane coated fine wire electrodes (0.08 mm in diameter) within a 60 mm long 23-gauge injection needle (0.65 mm in diameter) were inserted using the appliance (b) into the inferior head of the lateral pterygoid muscle. The tips of these fine wire electrodes were exposed 1 mm and bent 3 mm and 5 mm into a hook from the tip. After confirmation of correct placement of the fine wire electrodes, the appliance and needle were removed carefully.

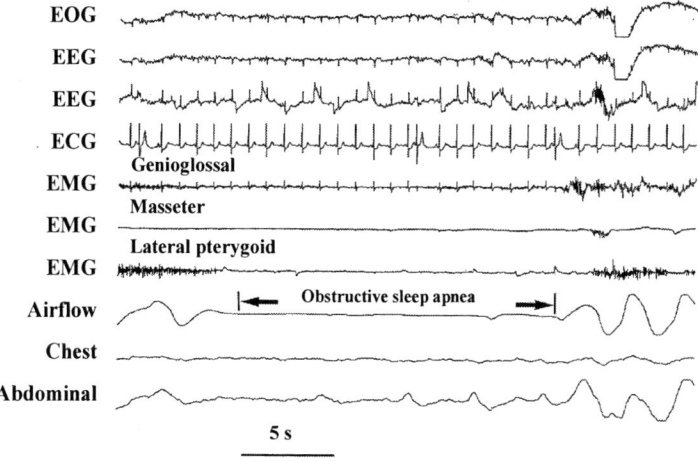

Figure 27. Polysomnographic recording during obstructive sleep apnea. During obstructive sleep apnea, airflow disappeared, but abdominal and chest movements remained partially. The genioglossal, masseter and lateral pterygoid muscles showed apparently reduced activity during obstructive sleep apnea.

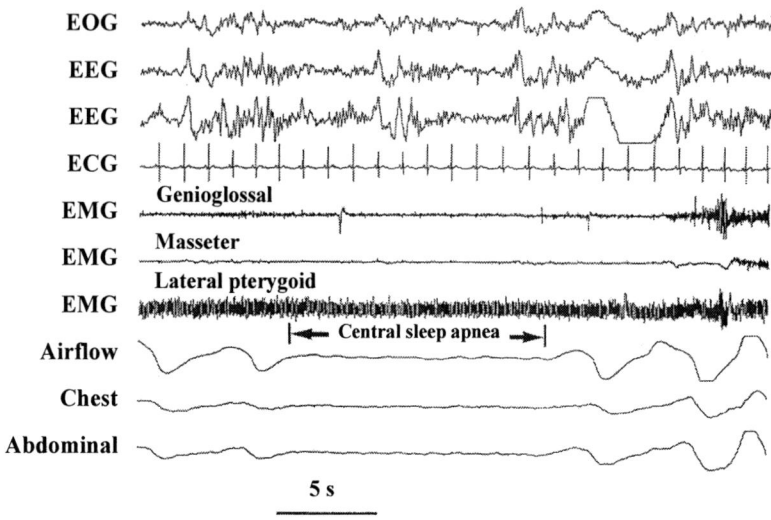

Figure 28. Polysomnographic recording during central sleep apnea. During central sleep apnea, both abdominal and chest movements disappeared completely, and the three muscles showed no obvious reductions.

On the other hand, during central sleep apnea, both abdominal and chest movements disappeared completely, and the three muscles showed no obvious reductions (Figure 28).

The muscles demonstrated significantly lower EMG amplitudes (genioglossal muscle, $p<0.0001$; masseter muscle, $p<0.005$; lateral pterygoid muscle, $p<0.005$) during than before obstructive apneas, and significantly higher EMG amplitudes (genioglossal muscle, $p<0.0001$; masseter muscle, $p<0.0001$; lateral pterygoid muscle, $p<0.0002$ after the apnea) (Figure 29).

The number of central apneic episodes per hour was low (1.7 ± 1.9). The central apnea index ranged from 0 to 6.4. No decrease in the mean EMG amplitude during central apneas was observed. The muscles showed significantly higher (genioglossal muscle, $p<0.002$; masseter muscle, $p<0.003$; lateral pterygoid muscle, $p<0.003$) EMG amplitudes after than during apneas.

After the placement of the appliance, EMG amplitude increased except for genioglossal muscle after obstructive and central apneas and during central apneas. The muscles exhibited significantly lower EMG amplitudes (genioglossal muscle, $p<0.0001$; masseter muscle, $p<0.01$; lateral pterygoid muscle, $p<0.005$) during obstructive apneas compared with before, and then significantly higher EMG amplitudes (genioglossal muscle, $p<0.0001$; masseter muscle, $p<0.02$; lateral pterygoid muscle, $p<0.02$) after the apneas (Figure 29).

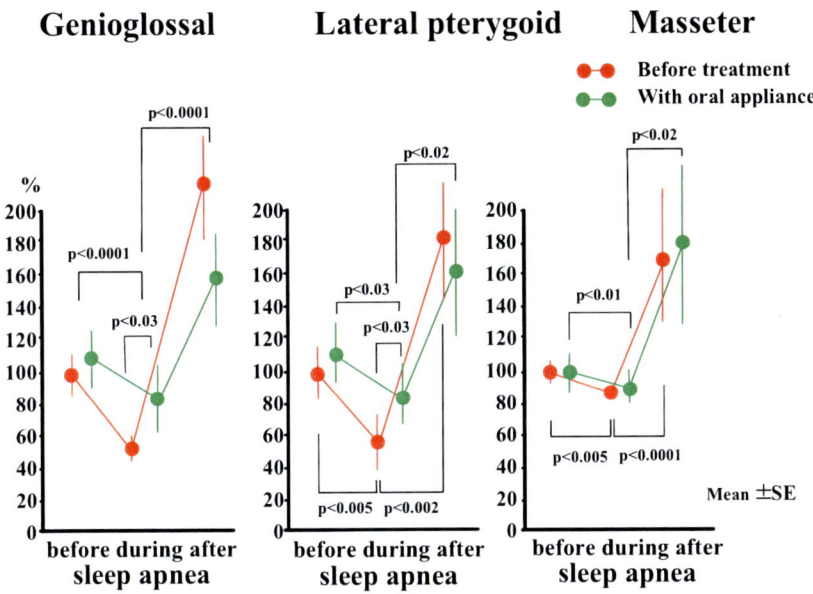

Figure 29. Relative muscle activity evaluated EMG activity before treatment as 100 %. The masseter muscle, the genioglossal muscle, and the inferior head of the lateral pterygoid muscle showed significantly lower electromyographic amplitudes during and higher amplitudes after obstructive apnea. The oral appliance helps maintain the tonus of the muscles by protracting the tongue and mandible even during sleep, which suggests that the activated muscles prevent the upper airway from collapsing (n=15).

No decrease in the mean EMG amplitude during central apneas was observed. The muscles demonstrated significantly higher EMG amplitudes after than during the apneas (genioglossal muscle, $p<0.02$; masseter muscle, $p<0.004$; lateral pterygoid muscle, $p<0.004$). The EMG amplitude of the genioglossal muscle during obstructive apneas ($16.9 \pm 5.8 \mu V$) was significantly increased ($p<0.03$) by the appliance ($27.6 \pm 18.8 \mu V$). Similarly, the lateral pterygoid muscle showed significantly higher EMG amplitude ($p<0.03$) during obstructive apneas with ($31.6 \pm 17.8 \mu V$) than without ($18.3 \pm 11.5 \mu V$) the appliance.

The patency of the upper airway is maintained normally by muscle tone and elasticity of the upper airway muscle. Remmers et al. [98] reported that genioglossal EMG of patients with SAS consistently revealed periodicity: low level activity at the onset of obstruction and prominent discharge at the instant of pharyngeal opening. Hollowell and Suratt [136] found that the masseter muscle was activated in patients with SAS in a manner similar to the submental muscles. Similarly, in the current study, the masseter muscle, the genioglossal muscle, and the inferior head of the lateral pterygoid muscle showed relatively low EMG amplitudes during and high EMG amplitudes after obstructive apnea.

The coactivation of agonist (the genioglossal and the lateral pterygoid muscle) and antagonist (the masseter muscle) after the apnea was postulated to stabilize the mandible to prevent the upper airway from collapsing. Muscles under the surface electrodes for the genioglossal muscle in this study can include the genioglossus, geniohyoid, mylohyoid, anterior belly of the digastric, and platysma. However, Sauerland et al.[137] reported that muscle activities during respiration can be followed closely by this surface recording during respiration. Hollowell and Suratt [136] reported that the mouths of patients with SAS opened wider than those of normal subjects at the end of expiration and further still at the end of inspiration, particularly at the termination of apneas when the masseter and submental muscles contracted. Morikawa et al. [138] investigated anesthetized, curarized subjects who were supine with their necks extended and observed that closing their jaws increased the mean distance between their tongue and posterior pharyngeal wall from 11 to 17.5 mm. The mouth opening at the end of expiration could narrow the upper airway, whereas opening at the end of inspiration could reflect the effort to expand the airway through tracheal tug and submental muscle activation that results in an opening of the mouth to allow mouth breathing. The hypotonia of the masticatory and tongue muscles and the weight of mandible, particularly in the supine position, can lead to opening of the mouth and further dorsal displacement of the mandible and tongue, resulting in pharyngeal narrowing and airway resistance, and finally obstructive apnea. The coactivation of elevator and depressor muscles after an apnea could stabilize the mandible to prevent the oropharynx from obstruction.

The EMG amplitudes of muscles increased after insertion of the appliance in this study. The results indicated that the device activates the muscles. The EMG amplitude of the genioglossal muscle during obstructive apnea was significantly increased by the appliance. The lateral pterygoid muscle showed significantly higher EMG amplitude during obstructive apneas with the appliance than without it. The results suggest that, during obstructive apneas, the tonus of the muscles protracting the tongue and mandible were maintained at an increased vertical and protrusive position. So relaxation of muscle contraction did not occur, which resulted in a significant increase in mean EMG amplitude during obstructive apnea. The activated muscles that protract the tongue and mandible prevented the upper airway from collapsing.

No reduction in the mean EMG amplitude was seen during central apneas. Thus, central apneas are suggested to occur independent of masticatory and tongue muscle activity. In other words, a central apnea can occur in the case of a loss of neural chest and abdominal respiratory drive even if the muscles are active and the upper airway is patent. After placement of the device, the EMG amplitude of the genioglossal muscle decreased during and after central apneas. No significant changes were observed even after inserting the appliance. Central sleep apnea is a disorder characterized by repeated apneic episodes during sleep that result from temporary loss of respiratory effort [139]. Central apnea differs from obstructive or mixed apneas by the absence of upper airway collapse and subsequent ventilatory attempts against an occluded airway. In most patients with central apnea, no obvious cause or association can be detected. Önal et al. [140] postulated that central apneas result from an abnormality in inhibition of the expiratory "off-switch" or inspiratory "on-switch" mechanism. P_{CO2} is the primary stimulus to ventilation during sleep and loss of this drive, as occurs with hypocapnia, may produce dysrhythmic breathing. Patients with complete absence of ventilatory chemosensitivity such as occurs with Ondine's curse (central alveolar hypoventilation) also have central apneas. Önal et al. [140] reported that, before the onset of a central apnea, the periodicity of diaphragmatic and genioglossal EMG disappeared for a few breaths, expiratory times gradually increased, and tracings of airflow and thoracoabdominal motion indicated that the apnea represents an extremely prolonged expiratory phase.

b. Movement-Related Cortical Potentials

Kornhuber and Deecke [141] (1965) first recorded a slowly increasing negative cortical potential called movement-related cortical potentials (MRCPs) beginning about 1 s before voluntary movements. The Bereitschaftspotential (BP proper), the negative slope (NS') and the motor potential (MP) are the main components of MRCPs for hand movement [142, 143]. BP proper is a gradually increasing, bilaterally widespread surface negativity with the maximum over the midline vertex region regardless of the site of movement, beginning about 1.5 s before the electromyographic (EMG) onset. It is followed by NS', which is a much steeper slope starting about 400 ms before the movement onset, and is characterized by a more localized negativity over the central and vertex areas contralateral to the movement [144]. This in turn is followed by MP, which is a small negative peak localized at the same region as NS', and starts at 50-60 ms before the EMG onset. MRCPs have been studied in association with the movements of finger, hand and foot, prior to biting [145], lip movements [146] and tongue protrusion [147]. In the present study we recorded MRCPs associated with deliberate open, close, right and left jaw movements to investigate the cortical mechanism underlying the control of human voluntary mandibular movement.

Ten healthy male subjects, aged 25 to 34 (average 30.6) years, and all right-handed according to the Edinburgh inventory [148] were evaluated in the present study. The order of opening, closing and lateral (right and left) movements was randomly selected. The subject sat in a comfortable chair, and was asked to make brisk movements (one of the four kinds of movements) at a self-paced rate of approximately once every 10 s, while fixating at a visual target placed about 1.5 m in front. The subject was trained before the experiment until each of the four movements could be performed satisfactorily for obtaining an accurate fiducial point. One of the four movements was repeated in succession until 50 trials were automatically recorded (EEGER, EEG Evoked response, Cambridge Electronic Design, U. K.). Then the next movement (one of the other three movements) was repeated similarly. After each of the four movements was recorded 50 times, the second session was held for each movement in the same fashion.

To confirm whether the subjects correctly performed the experimental movements, three-dimensional mandibular movements were recorded using a Mandibular Kinesiograph (MKG K6 Diagnostic System, Myo-tronics, Seattle, USA) [149, 150]. To detect the lateral preference of chewing, the subjects chewed one piece of gum, and visual inspections were made of either right or left side bolus placements [151]. In all subjects the preferential chewing side was the right. EMGs were recorded from the masseter muscle and the anterior belly of the digastric muscle on the right side using a pair of silver-silver chloride cup electrodes. Masseter EMG was used as the trigger point for mouth closing movement. Digastric EMG was used for mouth opening and lateral movements, because the lateral movement accompanies mouth opening, the anterior belly of the digastric is similarly activated [150, 151]. Electroencephalograms (EEGs) were recorded with 11 silver-silver chloride cup electrodes fixed on the scalp with collodion according to the International 10-20 System (F3, Fz, F4, T3, C3, Cz, C4, T4, P3, Pz and P4) with a band-pass filter of 0.05-100 Hz (BIOTOP 6R-12, San-ei, Japan). Each electrode was referred to linked ear lobe electrodes. Electrooculograms (EOGs) were recorded from an electrode placed at the lateral lower canthus of the right eye with reference to another electrode above the nasion.

All data were digitized with a sampling rate of 200 Hz and stored for off-line analysis. MRCPs for each session of each movement were obtained by averaging the EEG, using the EMG onset (the masseter muscle for closing movement, the digastric muscle for the other three movements) as the fiducial point (EEGER, EEG Evoked response, Cambridge Electronic Design, U. K.) [131]. Namely,

EEGs, EOGs and rectified EMGs were displayed on the screen, and the precise onset of the rectified EMG was visually determined and used as a trigger for back-averaging [152]. During this procedure, samples contaminated with artifacts such as eye movements or EMG were completely rejected. After confirming the reproducibility of waveforms among two like sessions of each movement by superimposing them on the computer, a group average waveform was obtained by averaging the data of those two sessions.

The EEG segments from 3.0 to 3.5 s prior to the EMG onset were averaged and used as a baseline for each channel. Amplitude of BP/NS' (BP and NS' combined together) at each electrode was measured from the baseline at the time of the EMG onset.

The onset of BP was determined by computer algorithm (EEGER, EEG Evoked response, Cambridge Electronic Design, U. K.) on the waveform obtained at Cz as the consistent take-off point from the baseline of a smoothed curve extrapolated from the raw data. The NS' onset was defined as the inflexion point of this curve to a steeper slope also at Cz.

Finally a grand average for each movement was obtained across all subjects. Topography of the cortical potentials was determined as isopotential maps using the grand average waveforms for each movement (Microsoft Excel®, Microsoft Corporation, USA).

The t-test with a Bonferroni correction and the analysis of variance (ANOVA) were used to assess the statistical significance of differences.

Grand average waveforms of MRCPs across all the subjects for each movement are shown in Figure 30.

Between 1.5 and 2.0 s preceding the EMG onset, a gradually increasing, bilaterally widespread negativity was observed diffusely with the maximum at the Cz electrode, although the onset of the potentials could not be clearly identified. The negative slope (NS') occurred 300-700 ms before the movement onset. The motor potential (MP) could not be assessed due to artifacts arising from the EMG of the masticatory muscles and movement artifacts just after the movement onset (Figure 31).

Figure 32 compares the mean BP/NS' amplitudes in the four kinds of movements, measured from the baseline at the Cz electrode at the EMG onset. Amplitude was significantly higher for the left lateral movement (6.1 ± 1.0 µV) than for mouth opening (3.8 ± 1.3 µV, $p<0.05$, ANOVA) and mouth closing (1.5 ± 1.7 µV, $p<0.002$, ANOVA). Mean amplitude for right lateral movement (5.3 ± 2.5 µV) was significantly higher than that for mouth closing ($p<0.008$, ANOVA).

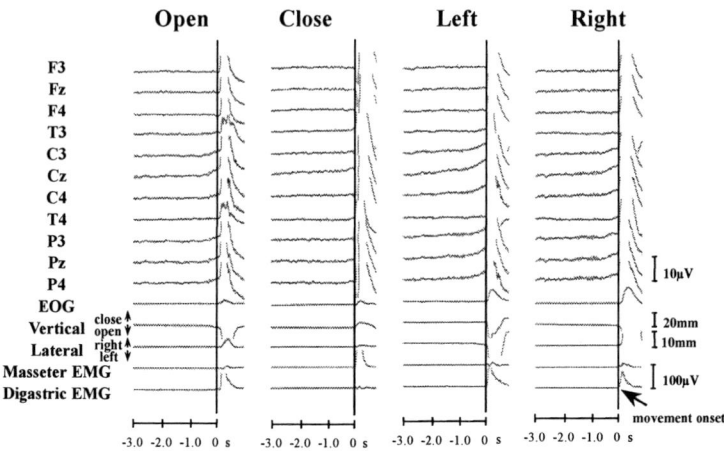

Figure 30. Grand average waveforms of movement-related cortical potentials (MRCPs) across all subjects (n=10) for four different kinds of voluntary movements, all involving the masticatory muscles. A gradually increasing, bilaterally widespread negativity is seen preceding the EMG onset, with the maximum at the Cz electrode for all four kinds of movements. Open: mouth opening, Close: mouth closing, Left: left lateral movement, Right: right lateral movement, MKG: Mandibular Kinesiograph, C: close, O: open, R: right, L: left.

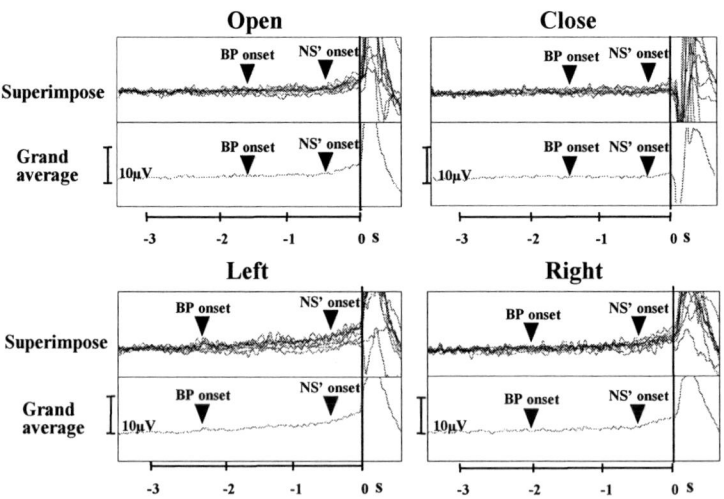

Figure 31. Superimposition and grand average waveforms of BP/NS' at Cz of all subjects (n=10) for each movement. The negative slope (NS') occurred 300-700 ms before the movement onset. The motor potential (MP) could not be assessed due to artifacts arising from the EMG of the masticatory muscles and movement artifacts just after the movement onset.

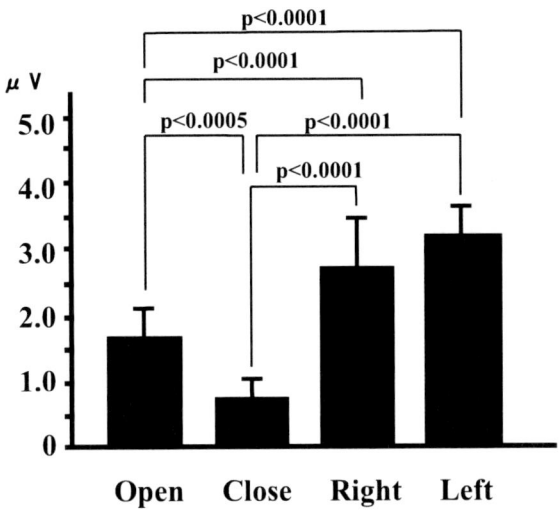

Figure 32. Mean BP/NS' amplitudes measured at Cz of all subjects (n=10) for each movement. Vertical bars indicate standard deviation. The mean BP/NS' amplitudes are significantly higher (ANOVA) for the left lateral movement (6.1 ± 1.0 µV) than for the mouth opening (3.8 ± 1.3 µV) and mouth closing (1.5 ± 1.7 µV), and that for the right lateral movement (5.3 ± 2.5 µV) is significantly higher (ANOVA) than for the mouth closing.

Figure 33 shows the mean BP/NS' amplitudes at all electrodes for each movement. The amplitude is maximum at Cz for all four kinds of movement. The topographic map of BP/NS' is shown in Figure 34. The isopotential map of BP/NS' for mouth opening and closing showed a symmetric distribution over the head. In contrast, that for the left lateral movement revealed a predominance in the left hemisphere; the mean amplitude at T3 (2.3 ± 1.5 µV) was significantly higher than that at T4 (0.5 ± 0.55 µV) (p<0.03, t-test). Right lateral movement showed higher amplitudes over the right hemisphere (0.81 ± 0.97 µV at T3 and 1.7 ± 1.2 µV at T4), although the difference did not reach statistical significance (p=0.25).

This study showed a gradually increasing, bilaterally widespread surface-negative potential preceding the voluntary, self-paced mandibular movements. Its amplitude reached a maximum over Cz. Very slow glossokinetic potentials as well as other speech muscle activities may resemble MRCPs, because these occur before the onset of tongue protrusions or vocalizations [153, 154]. Recent studies reported MRCPs in association with vocalization, by using methods carefully designed to exclude artifact contamination by speech muscle activities and glossokinetic potential [147, 155].

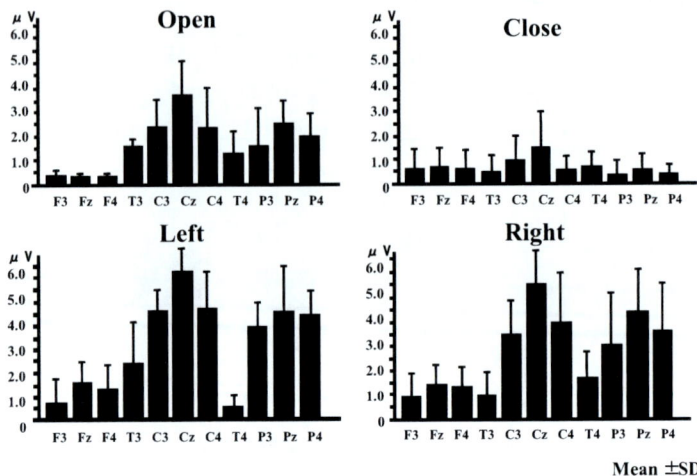

Figure 33. Mean BP/NS' amplitude at each electrode of all subjects (n=10) for the four kinds of movement. Vertical bars indicate standard deviation. The amplitudes are generally higher for the lateral movements than for the mouth opening or mouth closing, and the mouth closing shows the smallest amplitude. Each movement shows a symmetric distribution of BP/NS' with the maximum at the Cz electrode.

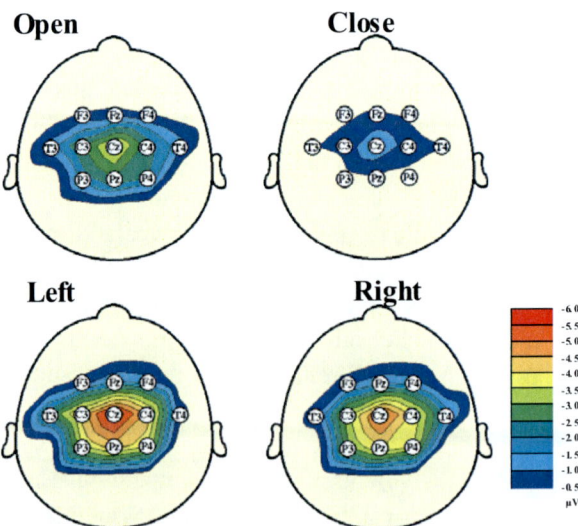

Figure 34. Isopotential maps of BP/NS' associated with four different kinds of movement of all subjects (n=10), all involving the masticatory muscles. The maps for the mouth opening and closing show a symmetric distribution over the head. In contrast, the maps for the lateral movements reveal a predominance over the hemisphere ipsilateral to the direction of movement, although the amplitude is maximum at Cz.

It is uncertain whether such artifacts are observed prior to mandibular movements. Ikeda et al. [147] proved the presence of MRCPs associated with tongue protrusion, recording artifact free potentials from chronically implanted subdural electrodes. The possibility of contamination by such artifacts was excluded in the present study.

Our results are comparable to MRCPs in association with finger, hand and foot movements, which consist of BP proper, NS' and MP [141]. The results obtained from subdural electrodes indicated that BP proper occurs in the bilateral hand primary and supplementary motor areas preceding unilateral hand movement, but later components (NS' and MP) become localized to the contralateral motor area [156]. In the present study, the topography of the whole pre-movement negative shift (BP/NS') in mouth opening and closing showed a bilaterally symmetric distribution. This is probably because the motor areas on both sides are active for this movement. Nakajima et al. [145] reported that the BP and NS' have been recorded prior to jaw biting and the amplitudes were largest (8-9 µV) in the ipsilateral temporal areas. But it is unclear whether the artifacts due to temporal EMG on the biting side could be perfectly excluded. The mouth closing in the current study was not biting, but closing from rest position to the intercuspal position. The amplitudes in the temporal areas were much smaller and the vertex region showed the highest amplitude. On the other hand, the map of BP/NS' for the lateral mandibular movements revealed a tendency of predominance over the ipsilateral hemisphere, although it was maximal at Cz. For the lateral mandibular movements, the inferior head of the lateral pterygoid muscle contralateral to the direction of movement pulls the condyle forward, downward and medially, while the ipsilateral posterior temporal muscle holds the ipsilateral condyle. The function of the lateral pterygoid is kinetic and isotonic, and that of the temporal muscle is tonic and isometric. This difference of activation might be responsible for the asymmetric amplitudes of BP/NS' at the temporal regions, although the precise mechanism is unknown. Despite the lack of significant difference, the mean amplitude of BP/NS' was higher in the left than in the right lateral movement. All the subjects in the present study showed right preferential chewing side, and it is likely that non-habitual left lateral movements required a longer preparatory period than did the preferential right lateral movements. Further experiments with firm control of movements are required to elucidate the mechanisms concerning differences of distribution and amplitude for lateral movements.

The amplitudes of negativity at movement onset were approximately 8-9 µV for biting movement [145], 5-6 µV for lip movement [146], 8-10 µV for finger movement [142], 10 µV for hand movement [141], 7-10 µV for vocalization [146,

155], and 10-15 µV for foot movement [141, 157]. The mean amplitudes of BP/NS' for the mouth opening and closing in this study were lower than those of other movements, and amplitudes for lateral movements were comparable to those for lip movement. Many studies have demonstrated that BP is influenced by the complexity of movement; the more difficult the task, the larger the amplitude of BP. The complexity of a movement may be related to the number of muscles and joints utilized [158], the sequence of activation [159, 160], the precision or attention [161], and the novelty or unfamiliarity of the movement to the subject. Mouth opening and closing are frequently used stereotyped movements as compared to finger or hand movements, which were previously used for MRCP recording. The lateral movements in this study were novel and far more unfamiliar to the subjects than finger or hand movements. Novelty or unfamiliarity may be an important factor that determined the BP/NS' amplitude in the present study. Familiar or semiautomatically performed movements such as mouth opening and closing are associated with smaller MRCP amplitudes, which implies more contributions from subcortical mechanisms as compared with those in novel movements.

This study demonstrated cortical potentials related to the basic, deliberately performed mandibular movements of opening, closing, right-lateral and left-lateral. The amplitude of these potentials in terms of the Bereitschaftspotential (BP proper) and the negative slope (NS') differed significantly between some of the movements. The BP/NS'-amplitudes for lateral movements were identical and tended to be larger than those for opening and closing. In addition, a tendency was seen for predominance in the ipsilateral hemisphere during right- and left-sided movements whereas the side-to-side distribution was symmetrical during opening and closing. However, further experiments with firm control of the magnitude and velocity of the different movements are needed to demonstrate the mechanisms and location of the underlying cortical control mechanisms [130].

c. Contingent Negative Variation

Contingent negative variation (CNV) is a long-latency event-related potential which develops in the interval between two stimuli, in which the first stimulus (S1) serves as a warning that prepares the subject to expect the second imperative stimulus (S2) which requires a decision or a motor response [162]. However, motor responses are not necessary to provoke the potentials, which occur during mere stimulus anticipation [163, 164]. It is assumed that CNV represents the neuronal activity necessary for sensorimotor integration or association and, therefore, is interpreted as an expression of the cognitive processes in preparation for a response directed to a purpose [162]. CNV consists of two components: a rapidly habituating early frontal component related to arousal and attention to the warning stimulus (S1), and a late component with a more central distribution [165]. The latter involves neural activities holding a motor response in readiness. The CNV is linked to different mental states and activities including arousal, stress, attention, expectation, level of vigilance, the will to elaborate a response, decisional performance, time estimation, and motor response preparation [166-168]. The frontal cortex has been considered as a likely generator for CNV in part because of its fronto-central scalp distribution, and the paradigm generating CNV is similar to memory tasks known to be dependent on the prefrontal cortex. Anterior cingulate gyrus, caudate nucleus, thalamus, and reticular formation may be crucial for the generation of the early CNV, and the dorsolateral prefrontal cortex may be involved in the generation of the late CNV [164]. Ikeda et al. [169], in a study with subdural recordings, stated that orbito-frontal and mesial frontal areas play an important role in regard to cognition and decision making. They reported that the basal ganglia are the most likely responsible for the generation of the late CNV [170]. Task-specific CNV amplitude loss was observed in patients with cervical dystonia [171] and writer's cramp [172]. The clinical symptom of dystonia may result from a deficient compensatory mechanism for abnormal motor programs in response to sensory stimuli [172, 173]. Reduced amplitude of movement-related cortical potentials has been reported in writer's cramp [174], torsion dystonia [174] and oromandibular dystonia [175]. These studies showed similar physiological abnormalities between other focal dystonia and oromandibular dystonia, suggesting a common pathophysiology [175]. It became of interest to clarify whether similar results in a cognitive paradigm would be found in oromandibular dystonia. So far, CNV has been studied mainly in association with the movements of the fingers, hands and feet. CNVs for various voluntary jaw and tongue movements and their cortical distribution have not been explored to our knowledge. In this study we examined CNVs associated with various jaw, tongue protrusion and hand extension tasks and compared the distribution and amplitude of the potentials among the movements to elucidate the motor control mechanism underlying mandibular and tongue movements.

We evaluated 10 healthy subjects (8 men and 2 women, ranging in age from 25 to 42 years with a mean of 34.4 years). They were all right-handed according to the Edinburgh inventory [148]. The warning signal (S1) was delivered using an apparatus, which was placed about 1 m in front of the subject and indicated 5 kinds of experimental movements by flashing 5 light emitting diodes. The upper light indicated mouth opening, lower light; mouth closing, left light; left lateral movement, right light; right lateral movement; middle light; tongue protrusion. These 5 signals were randomized but flashed with equal frequency on average. Two seconds after S1, a 1,000 Hz tone burst (S2) of 100 ms duration was delivered to both ears simultaneously through the earphones. The interval between S2 and the next S1 varied randomly between 4 and 7 s. During testing the subject sat in a comfortable reclining armchair with a head rest in a dimly lit, isolated and quiet room. The subject was asked to make the experimental movements from the jaw rest position as quickly as possible after hearing S2. To confirm whether the subjects performed the experimental movements correctly, three-dimensional incisal movements were recorded using a Mandibular Kinesiograph (MKG K6 Diagnostic System, Myo-tronics, Seattle, USA) [130, 176]. The right hand extension task was performed in the same fashion except for the S1. The subject was instructed to extend the right wrist after hearing the S2 irrespective of the 5 kinds of S1. The recording session for mandibular and tongue movements, and that for hand extension movements consisted of 150 and 30 trials respectively, and two sessions of each task were held interleaved by a rest period.

Electroencephalograms (EEGs) were recorded with a total of 19 surface tin cup electrodes (NeuroSoft, Inc. Virginia, USA) fixed on the scalp with gel according to the International 10-20 System (Fp1, Fp2, F7, F3, Fz, F4, F8, T3, C3, Cz, C4, T4, T5, P3, Pz, P4, T6, O1 and O2). Each electrode was referred to linked ear lobe electrodes. Electrooculograms (EOGs) were recorded with a pair of the same surface electrodes, one placed 2 cm above and the other 2 cm below the left canthus. EEG and EOG were recorded with a band-pass filter of 0.05-100 Hz. Electrode impedance was kept below 3 kΩ. Surface electromyograms (EMGs) were obtained with a band-pass filter of 0.05-100 Hz from a pair of tin cup electrodes placed on the skin overlying the masseter muscle (for mouth closing) and the suprahyoid muscles (for mouth opening, lateral movement and tongue protrusion) or the extensor digitorum communis muscle (for hand extension) on the right side. Suprahyoid EMG was used for lateral movement and tongue protrusion, since the movements accompany mouth opening, and the anterior belly of the digastric is similarly activated [149, 150].

All data were digitized with a sampling rate of 200 Hz and stored in a computer for off-line analysis (Scan™ 4.1, Neuroscan Labs, Inc. Virginia, USA). EEG data were averaged from 3 s before to 1 s after S2. The baseline was determined by averaging the 1 s epochs before the onset of S1. EEGs, EOGs and rectified EMGs were displayed on the screen. Samples contaminated with artifacts such as eye movements or EMGs were completely rejected. The grand average of CNVs for each task was obtained across all subjects by averaging the EEGs. The onsets of early and late CNVs were obtained as the inflexion points of waveforms to a more negative phase. The early CNV amplitude was defined as the mean value 500 ms after the S1 onset and late CNV amplitude as that at 1,900 ms after the S1 [172].

Statistical analysis was done by analysis of variance (ANOVA) with repeated measures design on the data using the following two factors: Task (six tasks) and Electrode (19 scalp sites). Task x Electrode interactions for early CNV and late CNV were examined with two-way ANOVA. To assess the significance in difference of amplitude at specific electrode positions, we used separate one-way ANOVA. The differences of these values were tested with a Tukey test.

The amplitudes of EMGs, EOGs and MKG showed no change after S1, indicating that the waveforms were not influenced by jaw and tongue muscle activities and their movement artifacts (Figure 35). After the S1, negative and positive peaks appeared with latencies of about 100 ms and 300 ms, respectively, and then a slowly increasing negativity was seen diffusely with the maximum in the vertex region (Figure 36, 37).

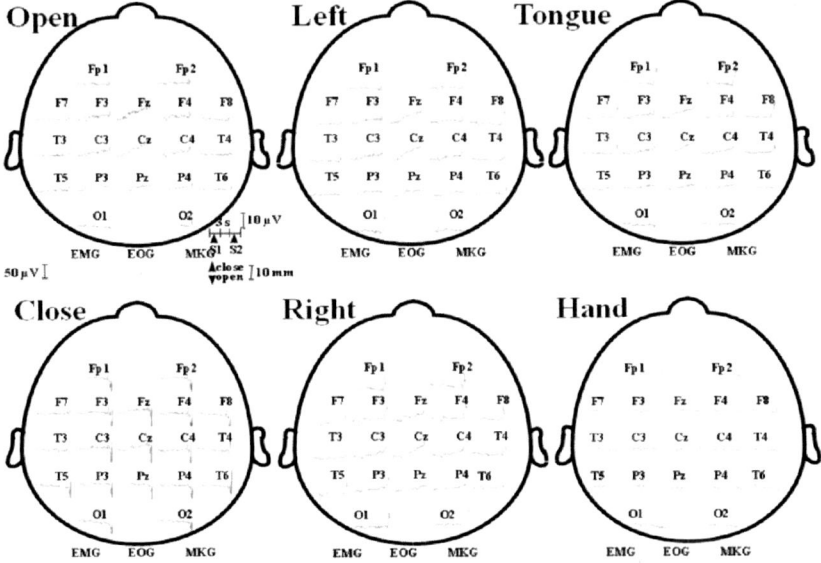

Figure 35. Grand average waveforms of contingent negative variations (CNVs) across all subjects for six different kinds of voluntary movements. A gradually increasing, bilaterally widespread negativity is observed, with the maximum in the vertex region for all tasks. Open: mouth opening, Close: mouth closing, Left: left lateral movement, Right: right lateral movement, Tongue: tongue protrusion, Hand: hand extension, EMG: masseter EMG for mouth closing, extensor digitorum communis EMG for hand extension, suprahyoid EMG for the other tasks, EOG: electrooculogram, MKG: Mandibular Kinesiograph.

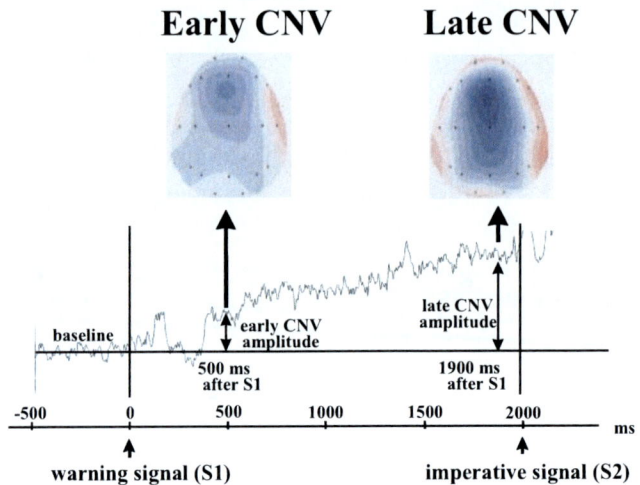

Figure 36. Early CNV and late CNV for mouth opening movement. The early CNV occurred 400-500 ms after S1. The late CNV was identified 1,000-1,200 ms after S1, and slowly increased until movement onset.

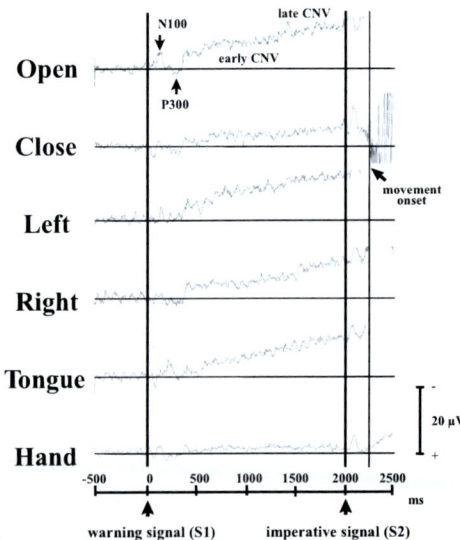

Figure 37. Grand average waveforms of CNVs at Cz (midline-central area) across all subjects for the six movements. The early CNV occurred 400-500 ms after S1. The late CNV was identified 1,000-1,200 ms after S1, and slowly increased until movement onset. After the onset, the potentials were contaminated with artifacts. Open: mouth opening, Close: mouth closing, Left: left lateral movement, Right: right lateral movement, Tongue: tongue protrusion, Hand: hand extension.

The early CNV was identified about 400-500 ms after the S1, mainly at the midline-frontal (Fz) and midline-central (Cz) areas (Figure 37). The late CNV started approximately 1000-1200 ms after the S1 and gradually increased until the S2 (Figure 37). After the movement onset, the potentials were contaminated with artifacts arising from the EMGs of the masticatory muscles and movement artifacts just after the movement onset.

The two-way ANOVA for early CNV disclosed significant interactions in Task x Electrode (F=91.42, p<0.0001, Task: F=84,03, p<0.0001, Electrode: F=1084.2, p<0.0001). The results of two-way ANOVA for late CNV showed significant Task x Electrode interaction (F=66.71, p<0.0001, Task: F=95.0, p<0.0001, Electrode: F=1253.83, p<0.0001).

The early CNV amplitudes measured at 500 ms after S1 were maximum at Fz (mean ± standard error, mouth opening: -8.0 ± 0.9 µV, mouth closing: -2.6 ± 0.7 µV, left lateral excursion: -8.5 ± 1.0 µV, right lateral excursion: -3.7 ± 0.6 µV, tongue protrusion: -3.0 ± 0.8 µV, hand extension: -1.5 ± 0.3 µV) (Figure 38). The mean amplitude at Fz was significantly lower for the hand extension (p<0.001, ANOVA) than for other jaw and tongue movements except mouth closing. The amplitude for the left lateral movement was significantly higher (p<0.001) than for mouth closing, right lateral movement and tongue protrusion tasks. The right lateral movement showed significantly higher (p<0.001) amplitude than those for mouth closing and tongue protrusion.

The late CNV amplitude measured at 1,900 ms after S1 was maximal at Cz (opening: -15.7 ± 2.1 µV, closing: -8.2 ± 1.3 µV, left: -17.1 ± 2.2 µV, right: -15.3 ± 1.9 µV, tongue: -12.5 ± 1.6 µV, hand: -3.1 ± 0.4 µV), and it was almost symmetrical (Figure 38). The mean late CNV amplitude at Cz was significantly higher (p<0.001) for the left lateral movement than for right lateral movement, tongue protrusion, mouth closing and hand extension. The mean amplitude was significantly lower for the hand extension task (p<0.001) than for the other movements. The late CNV amplitudes for right lateral movement and mouth opening were significantly higher (p<0.001) than mouth closing and tongue protrusion.

In general, the amplitudes were higher for lateral movements and mouth opening than for mouth closing, and the hand extension showed the smallest amplitude (Figure 38). The early CNV amplitude was maximum at Fz and the late CNV was maximum at Cz for all tasks, but the amplitude for the hand extension at the C3 showed almost the same amplitude as that at Cz (Figure 39). Slowly increasing bilaterally widespread negativities were observed starting after the S1 until movement onset after the S2 in the representative topographical maps (Figure 39).

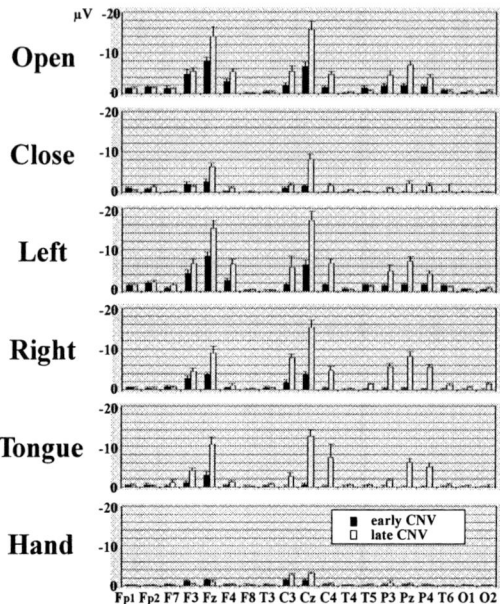

Figure 38. Mean CNV amplitudes at each electrode for the six movements. In general the amplitudes are higher for the lateral movements than for mouth closing, and the hand extension shows the smallest amplitude. Each movement shows a symmetrical distribution of CNV with the maximum at the Cz electrode. Shaded bars are early CNV, and open bars are late CNV. Bars and lines indicate the means and standard errors. Open: mouth opening, Close: mouth closing, Left: left lateral movement, Right: right lateral movement, Tongue: tongue protrusion, Hand: hand extension.

The isopotential map showed symmetrical distribution over the head with the maximum in the vertex region. However, the peak of negativity for the hand extension was distributed between C3 and Cz (Figure 39).

Glossokinetic potentials as well as muscle activities may contaminate the CNV, therefore, we recorded EMGs from the masseter and suprahyoid muscles by surface electrodes, which should have picked up any artifacts from the masticatory, tongue or facial muscles. Since the averaged EMG traces showed no such activities before the movement (Figure 35), contamination is unlikely in this study.

Although the exact generator of the CNV in humans is still unclear, multiple cortical and subcortical regions have been suggested to participate in the generation of the CNV [177]. The early CNV was believed to reflect an attention process in the frontal cortex [178].

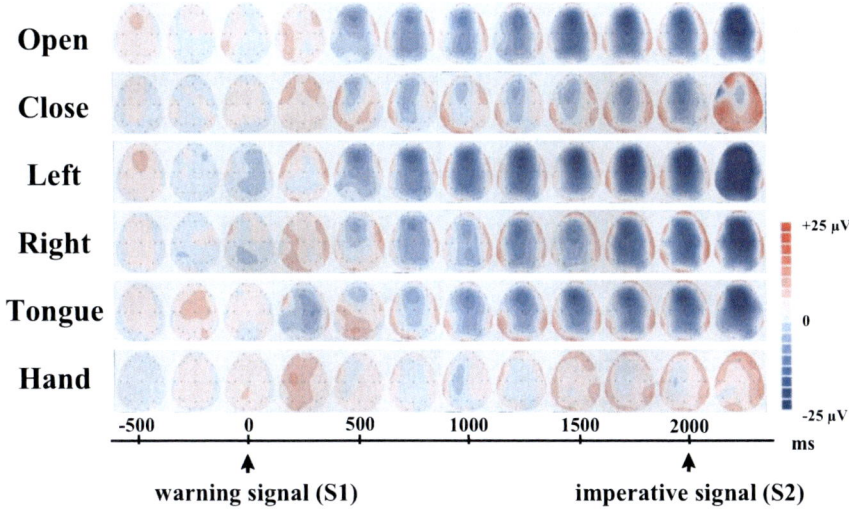

Figure 39. Scalp topography of the CNV for the six movements. The isopotential map of CNVs showed a symmetrical distribution over the head with the maximum in the vertex region. Each voltage scale is coded in blue for negative and red for positive. Open: mouth opening, Close: mouth closing, Left: left lateral movement, Right: right lateral movement, Tongue: tongue protrusion, Hand: hand extension.

The pre-frontal and parietal association cortices might be active in the judgment and decision-making process [179]. Cui et al. [180] suggested that there is an individual generator for the early CNV in the frontal lobe. A significant positive correlation between the amplitude of the early CNV and frontal cortex blood flow was reported [181]. The generators of the late CNV were found, using subdural recordings. They include supplementary, primary sensori-motor, pre-motor areas and pre-frontal cortex [177, 178, 182]. Further generator structures subdurally recorded in patients with epilepsy include the primary motor cortex, primary sensory area, supplementary motor area, basal pre-frontal, mesial pre-frontal, temporal and occipital regions [177, 182], and orbito-frontala and mesial frontal areas [169]. Cui et al. [180] suggested that the mesial wall motor areas as well as the primary motor cortexes and primary sensory areas participate in generating the late CNV, but these are not the only areas of generation for the late CNV.

The CNV amplitude may be affected by several factors including reaction times [162], the complexity of the task [183], the intensity of muscular effort [184], age [185] and mental status [186]. The amplitudes were -5-6 μV for hand movements [170, 187], -4.2 μV for finger extension [168] using a simple reaction time paradigm and -9 μV [172] using the S1 choice reaction paradigm. In a simple reaction time paradigm, the S1 and the task are always identical, while in the S1 choice paradigm, more than two kinds of S1 are delivered and the subject performs tasks according to the S1. The CNVs recorded with a simple reaction time paradigm suffered substantial effects of habituation in their amplitudes [171]. The CNV amplitudes for jaw and tongue movements in this study were higher than those already reported values for mouth opening and vocalization (-10-13 μV) [188, 189], which were performed using a simple reaction time paradigm. On the other hand, the amplitude for hand extension tended to be smaller than that reported previously [170, 187]. This discrepancy is possibly due to the different paradigm employed, because considerable variation in CNVs recorded with different paradigms has been reported [179]. In this study the subjects had to decide and prepare for one of the 5 tasks from the placement of the light, while the hand extension was executed similarly for all 5 kinds of S1. The subjects may have paid more attention to the jaw and tongue movements than the hand extension. The map of the movement-related cortical potentials, which begin about 1 s before a self-paced voluntary movement [141] measured at the movement onset for the lateral mandibular movements revealed predominance over the ipsilateral hemisphere to the direction of the movement [130]. In this study, however, all the jaw and tongue movements showed almost symmetrical distribution. The tendency of predominance over the hemisphere for lateral excursion may be overshadowed by the CNV potential, although the late CNV amplitude can involve a part of the movement-related cortical potentials. The map of CNVs for hand movement in this study showed a peak between C3 and Cz. CNV amplitudes were asymmetric, with left hemisphere dominance for right hand movement using the simple reaction time paradigm [171]. In a study using the S1 choice reaction paradigm, however, the difference was significant [172]. This discrepancy may be due to the different paradigms.

Bilateral CNV associated with jaw opening was recorded at several cortical locations, with a tendency for larger amplitudes at temporal placements [188]. In this study, however, as clearly shown in Figure 35, CNV for mouth opening revealed bilaterally spread negativity with the maximum at Cz. No remarkable amplitude was detected by the electrodes at temporal areas. The possibility that the potential at the temporal region was contaminated with temporal muscle EMG in the previous study could not be completely excluded. The maximal negativity recorded over the scalp from Cz in the present study is considered to reflect the activity of the supplementary motor area. The primary motor area for the jaw and tongue movements is thought to be located in the temporal areas, due to the orderly representation of the body within the precentral gyrus. Recently, a study using functional magnetic imaging with simultaneous CNV recording confirmed contributions from the supplementary area, cingulated, thalamus, and bilateral insula in anticipatory attention and motor preparatory processes engendered by the task that are indexed electrophysiologically by generation of the CNV [190]. The maximal negativity found presently is probably due to potentials from multiple cortical generators being summated at Cz through volume conduction. The scalp-recorded late CNV and Bereitschaftspotential (the main component of movement-related cortical potentials) have common cortical generators, but the underlying generating mechanism at the subcortical level may differ: the cortico-basal ganglia-thalamocortical circuit is responsible for the late CNV while the cortico-cerebello-cortical circuit produces the Bereitschaftspotential [170]. The more difficult the task, the larger the amplitude of the Bereitschaftspotential [191]. The amplitudes of movement-related cortical potentials are significantly higher for the lateral excursion of the jaw than for mouth opening and closing [130, 175]. Familiar or semiautomatically performed movements such as mouth opening and closing are associated with smaller amplitudes, which implies more contribution from subcortical mechanisms compared with those in unfamiliar tasks [130, 175]. The maximal CNV amplitude in this study was highest for the left lateral movement and lowest for mouth closing. The amplitude was higher for mouth opening than for right lateral movement, but not significantly. The reason for this difference remains uncertain. Further experiments with firm control of the direction, magnitude and velocity of the movements are needed to clarify the difference and the underlying control mechanism. Based on the similarity of the late CNV to Bereitschaftspotential related to the familiarity of tasks in this study, it may be that the two potentials share at least some cortical generators in common. The basal ganglia are most likely responsible for the generation of the late CNV and cerebellar efferent system for the generation of the Bereitschaftspotential [170].

Kaji et al. [171] recorded CNV in patients with cervical dystonia, by using neck and hand movements, as motor tasks in response to the imperative stimulus. They found a task-specific abnormality; the patients had significantly decreased late CNV amplitudes for head rotation, but not for finger extension. Dystonia is defined as a syndrome of sustained muscle contraction that frequently causes twisting and repetitive movements or abnormal postures. Hamano et al. [172] found significantly decreased CNV amplitudes for finger extension movement in patients with writer's cramp, a form of focal dystonia. Based on these findings, they proposed that cervical dystonia and writer's cramp are associated with defective retrieval or retaining of specific motor programs. Oromandibular dystonia is a focal dystonia manifested by involuntary masticatory and/or lingual muscle contraction [192, 193]. It is likely that similar results in a cognitive paradigm would be found in oromandibular dystonia. Reduced amplitude of movement-related cortical potentials was reported in oromandibular dystonia, suggesting the common pathophysiology and similar physiological abnormalities between other focal dystonia and oromandibular dystonia [175, 194]. CNV recording might be important for elucidating the neuronal activity necessary for the sensorimotor integration and pathophysiology of diseases with abnormal orofacial movements such as oromandibular dystonia or dyskinesia [131] and also SAS (Figure 40).

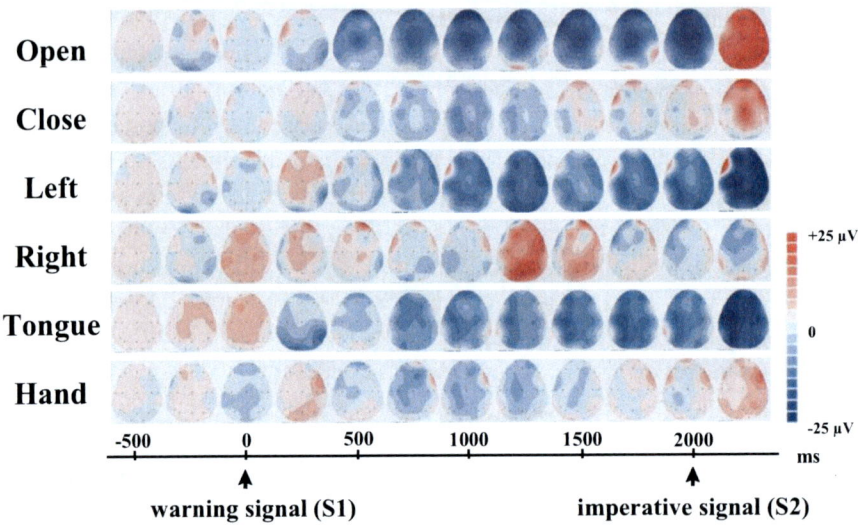

Figure 40. Scalp topography of the CNV for the six movements in a patient with SAS. The pattern of the isopotential map differs from that of normal control. The difference might be related to sleepiness due to SAS.

2. MAGNETOENCEPHALOGRAPHY

Brain imaging techniques such as positron emission tomography and functional magnetic resonance imaging (MRI) reflect cortical function by showing alterations in regional cerebral blood flow in the order of seconds that are secondary consequences of electric activity in the order of milliseconds, and thus have poor temporal resolution. Magnetoencephalography (MEG) offers excellent spatial and temporal localization of excited cortical areas in the order of millimeters and milliseconds.

It is well known that the primary somatosensorimotor cortex is organized in an orderly somatotopic way, which has been termed the "homunculus" representation of brain areas related to the whole human body [195]. The somatotopic organization for the oral organs in the primary somatosensory cortex (SI) has been studied by direct electric stimulation of the cortical surface [195], by intracranial recording of somatosensory evoked potentials (SEPs) [196] and of somatosensory evoked magnetic fields (SEFs) [197-204], and by functional MRI [205-207]. Although the general somatotopic organization indicates superior and medial location of the lip SI to the tongue SI, the mapping data show large interindividual variability. For example, the first mapping by Penfield and Rasmussen showed that the upper lip area was indicated superior to the lower lip area [195]. Some SEF studies suggested that the upper lip SI is superior to the lower lip SI [199-201], while both patterns of arrangement were observed in other studies [198, 202].

Obstructive sleep apneas are accompanied by collapse of the upper airway during sleep. The degree of collapse is indicated by the size of the pharyngeal lumen, which depends on the balance between the airway suction pressure and the tonus of upper airway dilator muscles such as the genioglossus. The long-term effects of severe sleep respiratory disturbances could result in dysfunction of the cortico-motoneuronal system [208]. Patients with SAS and habitual snorers exhibit an increased number of various nerve endings in the mucosal epithelium, which supports the hypothesis that the patients have a neurological disorder involving afferent fibers originating from the palatal mucosa [209, 210]. Snoring vibration occurring every night could cause local nerve damage in the soft palate, which could result in gradual airway collapse due to impairment of the reflex mechanism. Although disturbance of perception in the soft palate caused by local nerve damage has been reported in patients with SAS [211, 212], no study has dealt with the relevant responses in the central nervous system.

Recordings of SEFs allow noninvasive assessment of the functions of human somatosensory pathways. Air-puff stimulation selectively activates rapidly adapting cutaneous mechanoreceptors and is therefore suitable for studies of cortical areas involved in the processing of tactile stimuli [213]. Thus, to investigate the normal physiological mechanism of the perception of the tactile sensation in the soft palate, we measured the SEF following air-puff stimulation in healthy subjects [132].

We evaluated 7 healthy subjects (5 men and 2 women, age ranging from 26 to 41 years, with mean 34.4 years) in this study. Mean body mass index was 21.4 ± 2.0 kg/m^2 [18.3-24.2] (±SD [range]). Mean Epworth Sleepiness Scale was 3.7 ±

2.1 (2-7). None of the subject presented any history or symptoms related to respiratory disturbance during sleep.

An intraoral appliance was fabricated individually using copolyester foil (Erkodur, Erkodent, Pfalzgrafenweiler, Germany) on a maxillary cast (Figure 41).

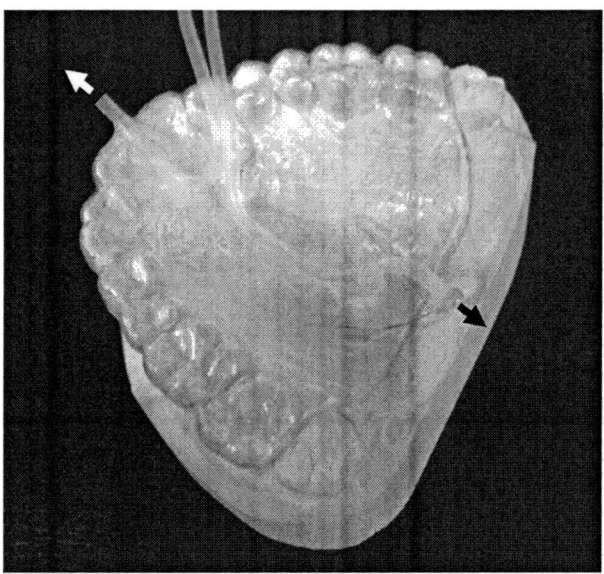

Figure 41. An intraoral device with two nozzles for soft palate air-puff stimulation. One nozzle is directed to the middle of the soft palate (black arrow) and the other is directed forward out of the mouth so as not to contact any part inside the mouth (white arrow). The air-puffs are produced by delivery of compressed nitrogen randomly to one of the two nozzles.

Two nozzles with inner diameter of 1 mm were attached to the device made of autopolymerizing resin (Quick Resin, Shofu, Kyoto, Japan). One nozzle was directed to the middle of the soft palate to maintain a constant distance (3 mm) from the stimulated mucosa and the other was directed forward out of the mouth so as not to contact any part inside the mouth.

The air-puffs were produced using compressed nitrogen using a Tactile Stimulator (NKP, Yokohama, Japan), and then passed through polyvinylchloride tubing (diameter 6 mm) randomly to one of the two nozzles (stimulation intensity, 70 kPa; stimulus duration, 100 ms; interstimulus interval, 1~2 s). The time delay from the trigger to the onset of air-puff at the outlet of the nozzle was 20 ms. Timing measurement for the magnetic field response was made from the onset of the air-puff assuming that there was delay of 20 ms.

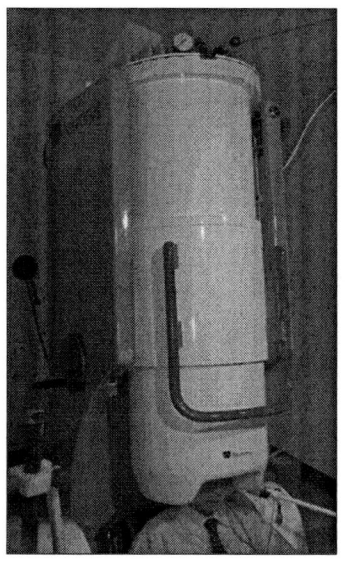 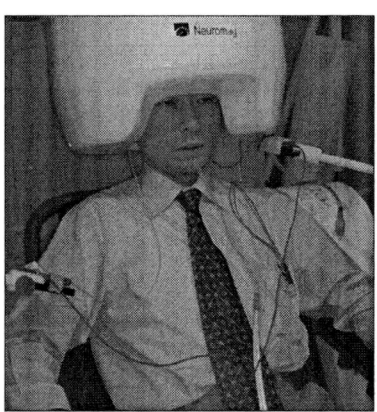

Figure 42. The somatosensory evoked magnetic field (SEF) was measured by using a helmet-shaped 122-channel neuromagnetometer with placement of the appliance in a shield room.

All subjects reported clear tactile sensations at the stimulated areas. The appliance in which the nozzles of the air-puffs were directed to the middle of the soft palate and forward out of the mouth (Figure 41) was used during the experiment. In order to mask the noise produced by the air-puffs, binaural white noise (75-80 dB SPL) was used, under which subjects could not hear the onset of air-puff stimulation.

The neuromagnetic signals were measured with a helmet-shaped 122-channel neuromagnetometer (Neuromag 122, Neuromag, Finland) in a magnetically shielded room (Figure 42). In this device, 61 pairs of two orthogonally oriented figure-of-eight first-order planar gradiometers detect the two orthogonal derivatives of the radial component of the magnetic field at each pair of locations [214], and typically detect the largest signal just above the corresponding generator source. Head position with respect to the sensor array was measured with head position indicator coils placed on defined scalp sites. The positions of head position indicator coils in relation to anatomical landmarks of the nasion and bilateral preauricular points, where oil tablets were placed for the MRI scanning, were measured with a 3D digitizer (Isotrak 3S1002, Polhelmus Navigation Sciences, Colchester, VT) to allow alignment of the MEG and MRI coordinate systems. We averaged separately the responses to the air-puff stimuli to the middle of the soft palate and those to the air-puff driven out of the mouth with the appliance (Figure 41). The recording band pass was 0.03-320 Hz for MEG, and the sampling rate for digital conversion was 970 Hz. The analysis window for averaging was 50 ms before to 500 ms after each trigger signal, namely 70 ms before to 480 ms after the onset of air-puff stimulation. Epochs containing MEG signals exceeding 1500 fT/cm were excluded automatically from the averaging. At least 200 of each of these stimuli were averaged for one session, and two sessions were held, with a rest period between sessions. To avoid any effects related to startle responses, averages were initiated after at least ten stimuli were given. In order to maintain the vigilance of the subjects, short breaks were given between the sessions. Continuous MEG waveforms from the occipital area were monitored to check the vigilance during measurements. Head MRIs were obtained with a 0.2 T Signa Profile System (General Electric Medical System, Milwaukee, USA) from all subjects.

A response was defined as when the signal exceeded the range of the resting activity (mean ± 2 SDs of the activity before 50 ms till the trigger pulse) [215]. The peak latency of the first response was measured from the channel showing the maximal signal. Isocontour maps were constructed at selected time points within the analysis window, using the minimum-norm estimate. The sources of the magnetic fields were modeled as equivalent current dipoles (ECDs), whose location, orientation and current strength were estimated from the measured magnetic waveforms. To identify the source of ECDs, the spherical head model whose center best fitted the local curvature of the subject's brain surface was adopted, based on the individual MRI [216]. We accepted only ECDs attaining 85% goodness-of-fit and confidence volume <1000 mm^3. Using the paired t-test, we compared statistically the peak latency and dipole moment of the middle and right side of soft palate stimulation with the second appliance.

In the recordings obtained with the device, in all 7 subjects, responses were observed symmetrically in the bilateral parietotemporal regions, with peak latency of about 130 ms from the soft palate stimulation at the middle portion. No distinct responses were observed in any of the subjects after control stimulation which was directed forward out of the mouth (Figure 43). Prior to this peak, no distinct early responses were observed. The peak latency was 126 ± 30 ms for the left and 127 ± 24 ms for the right hemisphere from the stimulation of the middle part of the soft palate (Figure 43) with the appliance. Estimation of ECD could not be accomplished in one subject because of unsuccessful measurement by the 3D digitizer. Another subject showed too weak a response to provide reliable ECD. Therefore, we were able to estimate ECDs for 5 subjects. The ECDs were located in the parietal region bilaterally and directed posteriorly (Figure 44).

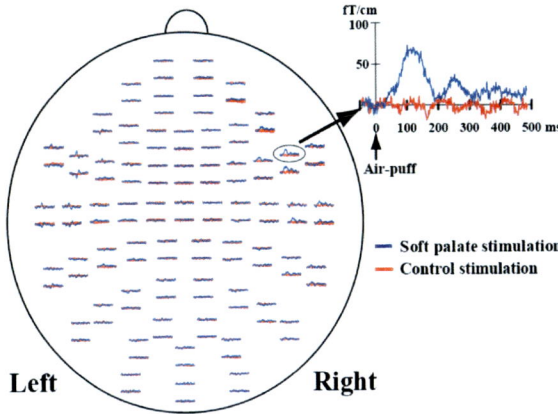

Figure 43. Waveforms of the SEF for the middle of the soft palate in a typical example (subject 1). The top view of the 122-channel recording shows large responses over the bilateral temporal areas. The traces are the average of 200 responses. Each trace started 50 ms before and ended 480 ms after a stimulus. As shown in the expanded waveforms, responses to soft palate air-puff stimulation (blue line) with an amplitude of about 60 fT/cm were identified symmetrically in the bilateral temporal region with a mean peak latency of 120 ms after the stimulation. No distinct responses were observed after control air-puff stimulation (red line).

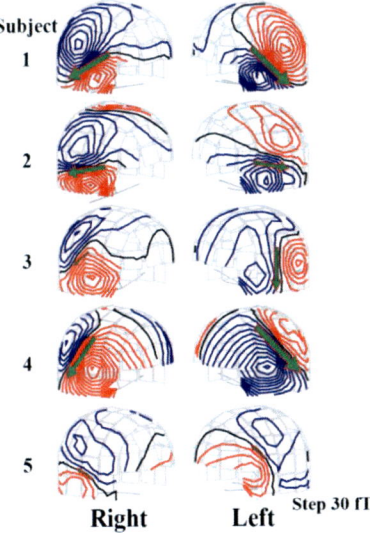

Figure 44. Isocontour maps obtained from the SEF for the middle of the soft palate 130 ms after the air-puff stimulation in 5 subjects. Red and blue lines indicate outgoing and ingoing fluxes, respectively. Green arrows show the location and direction of equivalent current dipoles producing the SEF distribution. Arrowheads indicate the negative pole.

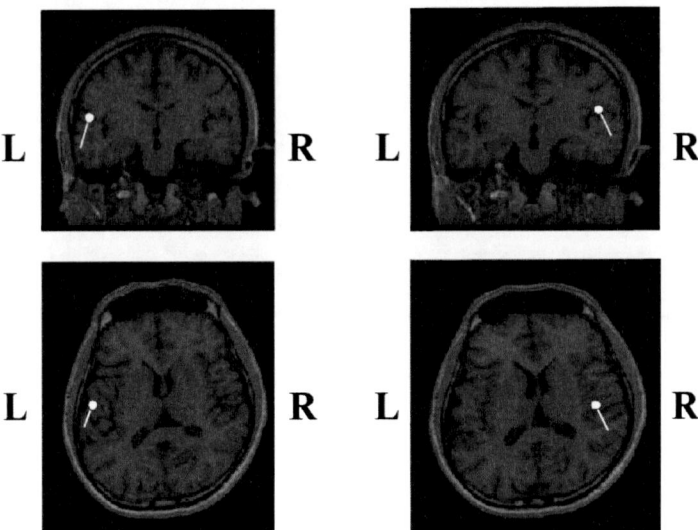

Figure 45. Equivalent current dipoles (ECDs) of the SEF for the middle of the soft palate 130 ms after the stimulation superimposed on the magnetic resonance images in a typical example (subject 1). On 9 hemispheres of 5 subjects, the corresponding ECD was estimated around the Sylvian fissure, the second somatosensory area. Circles and bars indicate equivalent current dipole location and orientation, respectively.

The dipole moment was 24.4 ± 9.9 nAm and 20.2 ± 7.6 nAm on the left and right hemispheres, respectively.

In 4 out of 5 subjects, ECDs were localized around the Sylvian fissure bilaterally, in the second somatosensory area (SII) (Figure 45). In the other subject (subject 5 in Figure 44), although the ECD was detected around the Sylvian fissure on the right side, it was located in the prefrontal area on the left side.

Long-latency responses were identified symmetrically in the bilateral parietal regions with a peak latency at approximately 130 ms from the onset of stimulation, while no distinct responses were detected after control stimulation directed forward out of the mouth. The responses were thought to be related not to an auditory reaction to noise produced by the air-puff output, but to tactile stimulation of the soft palate on the following grounds. First, the air-puff was masked with white noise. Second, the air-puff for control stimulation produced the same noise, but caused no response. In 9 hemispheres of 5 subjects, the ECDs were estimated around the Sylvian fissures, the SII. There was no significant difference between the results of the peak latency and dipole moment for the stimulation of the middle and right side of the soft palate. Since they did not show a clear hemispheric difference regarding the strength of the ECD even with right side stimulation, these responses can be regarded as being derived from SII. The number of subjects might not have been sufficient in this study, and a further study with a larger number of subjects may be warranted to draw conclusions regarding normal subjects. This method can provide important information on neurophysiological basis of upper airway perception [132].

Any difference in response between normal subjects and patients with sleep related respiratory disturbances may offer new insight into the pathogenesis of the condition. Hashimoto (1999) [213] studied the SEPs elicited by air-puff stimulation using a specially fabricated high-speed air-control system in which velocity and force could be varied. He reported that the peak latency of the initial component from air-puff stimulation of the tip of the index finger was slightly longer than that of electric SEPs, and that the amplitudes of SEP components were essentially similar for the two types of stimulation [213]. However, these findings might be true only for the special air-puff system. The difference between that system and the air-puff system in this work is unclear. Electric stimulation has been used in previous studies concerning palatal SEPs [196, 217]. The advantage of natural air-puff stimulation over electric stimulation is that the former produces a physiological pattern of stimulation of the afferent pathway, which can be generated by stimulating mechanoreceptors [213]. Air-puff stimulation should be more suitable than electric stimulation for the purpose of exploring the cortical reaction in response to natural tactile stimuli given to the soft palate. The ECD location was not detected in all subjects because the results did not meet our criteria for reliable ECD location. This might be due to the fact that air-puff stimulation is not as sharp and strong, and has inferior time-locking, compared to electrical stimulation [204].

Until now, no SEP studies have dealt with the response to soft palate stimulation in humans. Among the previous SEP studies involving stimulation in the oral cavity, electric stimulation of the greater palatine nerve showed peak latency similar to the N13 and P18 recorded in SEP to the lip [218]. Electric stimulation in the hard palate induced responses in the somatosensory cortex just superior to the Sylvian sulcus, as shown by the intracranial recording of SEPs [196]. These responses had positive peaks at 20-40 ms and 100-130 ms, and a negative peak at 50-70 ms. However, the same authors suggested the possibility that electric stimulation of the hard palate might have elicited tooth and gum afferents simultaneously [218]. The above-mentioned studies indicate the difficulty of using electric stimulation of the hard palate without activating other parts of the oral cavity. In our study, the recorded responses must have had little influence from the activation of other parts, since we directed the air-puff to the middle of the soft palate.

In this study, we could not detect an early reaction to air-puff stimulation of the soft palate. Why no distinct cortical responses were observed remains uncertain. One possibility is that the air-puff stimulation in the present study might not be suitable for evoking the early reaction. The recorded responses were relatively small. It is difficult to detect smaller brain activation of horizontally oriented dipoles or those radial to the skull. Possibly, we could not record such small or radially-oriented responses if there were any. Usually, the primary response can be elicited only when the stimuli are synchronized in time. Another possibility is that the early response might be absent for stimulation of the soft palate. McCarthy and Allison [218] postulated that the most lateral portion of the postcentral gyrus may contain the representation of posterior intraoral structures. However, it was not possible for them to detect the responses for the soft palate and pharynx by electric stimulation with cortical surface recording in monkeys even though it covered the most lateral portion of the gyrus, at least using their recordings made up to 80 ms after the stimulation. Therefore, it seems reasonable to assume the absence of an early response to soft palate stimulation in humans.

The SII is located along the superior bank of the Sylvian fissure, and lies lateral and inferior to the face representation in the SI. One of the major advantages of SEFs is the capability of detecting activity in the SII. SEF responses to electric stimuli to the lip from SII peaked 90-110 ms after stimuli in the bilateral SII [198, 219]. SII responses to contra- and ipsilateral stimuli were almost symmetric for face stimulation and clearly asymmetric for hand stimulation [197]. In this study, the responses to the middle and right side of the soft palate stimulation were almost identical and distributed bilaterally and symmetrically. This would be a characteristic of the reaction derived from the SII. Since the results of the middle and right side stimulation did not show clear laterality regarding the strength of the ECD, these responses could be regarded as being derived from the SII. However, bilateral activation of SEF was evident at trigeminal areas [198]. Moreover, the sites of stimulation by air-puffs to the middle and right side of the soft palate can overlap to some degree. Therefore, it is uncertain from the findings of this study whether the origin of the reaction was the SI or SII.

Both painful and nonpainful mechanical stimulation or electric stimulation of visceral esophageal afferents can elicit SII responses bilaterally, but there is no clear SI activation [220, 221]. This suggests that the SII is the primary activated area after esophageal stimulation and presumably also following other visceral stimulation [220] and that the visceral afferents lack a significant SI representation [221]. Both noxious and visceral stimuli may activate the SII cortices directly [222]. Although it is impossible to draw a conclusion from the results of this study, tactile afferents from the soft palate might primarily project to the SII and lack a significant SI representation. Further studies using intracranial recording will be necessary to confirm this hypothesis.

In conclusion, we could record responses with peak latency of about 130 ms to air-puff stimulation of the soft palate in the bilateral second somatosensory areas. This method can provide important information about the neurophysiological basis of upper airway perception (Figure 46).

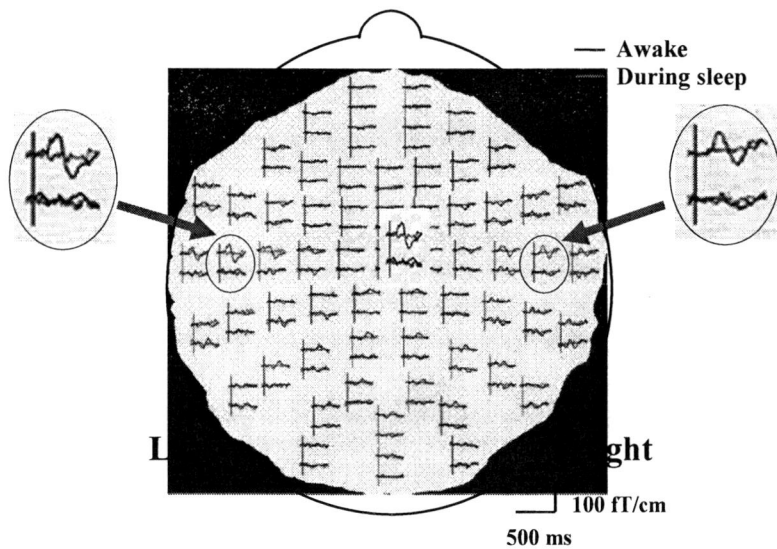

Figure 46. Waveforms of the SEF for the middle of the soft palate during sleep. The responses apparently reduced after falling asleep.

3. NEAR-INFRARED SPECTROSCOPY

Recent advances in functional brain-imaging techniques such as positron emission tomography (PET), functional magnetic resonance imaging (fMRI), and magnetoencephalography (MEG) have enabled examination of brain activity during various tasks. PET study requires intravenous injection of oxygen-15-labelled water as a tracer, and the spatial and temporal resolution is low. It has been considered difficult to obtain satisfactory fMRI during jaw movements because the head motion during jaw movements causes artifacts on the images.

PET and fMRI reflect changes in cortical function that are secondary consequences to alterations in regional cerebral blood flow, and have poor temporal resolution. MEG allows excellent spatial and temporal localization of excited cortical neurons in the order of millimeter and millisecond, but mappings of regional brain activity during various oral function such as chewing or clenching are difficult to record because of artifacts resulting from head and jaw movement and masticatory or facial muscle activity.

Neither MEG nor EEG could be discerned due to artifacts arising from the EMG of the masticatory muscles and to movement artifacts just after the movement onset. Brief orofacial movements that induce artifacts may be problematic in fMRI [223]. Moreover, such movement could produce an activation-related signal if the movement was correlated with the activation condition.

Near-infrared spectroscopy is a non-invasive technique which permits the measurement of cerebral blood volume and oxygen saturation in response to brain activation through the intact skull [224, 225]. Since flexible optical fibers connecting the examinee and the main unit make it easy to test, this tool has great advantages in compensating for subject movement.

To evaluate the differences in brain activity with SAS, we measured functional brain imaging of cerebral blood volume with various tasks in SAS patients by multi-channel near-infrared spectroscopy. The Hitachi ETG-100 Optical Topography (Hitachi Medical, Tokyo, Japan) device is used to record brain activity in optical properties of brain tissue simultaneously from 24 channels. It can estimate the changes in the concentration of oxyhemoglobin (oxy-Hb), deoxyhemoglobin (deoxy-Hb) and total hemoglobin (total-Hb) in response to stimulation with 0.1 -second time resolution [226].

Channels mostly measure vascular changes from the surface of the cortex below the scalp. The imaging of reflected light as a measure of neural activity has widespread use in the study of functional architecture of the cortex [227]. Figure 47 shows a schematic mechanism of the optical topography. We evaluated relative change in total-Hb, which means blood volume, from an arbitrary zero baselines at the start of the measurement period on the basis of Lambert–Beer law [228]. The exact optical path length of the light traveling through the brain tissue was not known, the unit of these values was molar concentration multiplied by length (mMol·mm). We placed a pair of 3 x 3 arrays with five incident and four detection fibers. The probes of the optical topography were attached to the bi-lateral temporal area cortex (Figure 47).

Subjects were allowed to determine their own most comfortable posture. And then the probes of the optical topography were mounted on a flexible cap, over the right and left temporal areas of each subject's head (Figure 47).

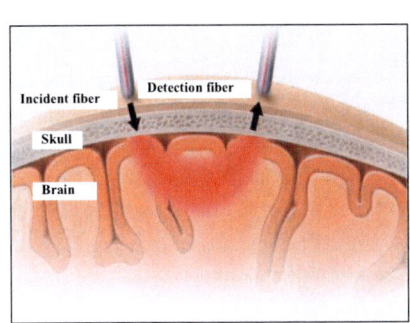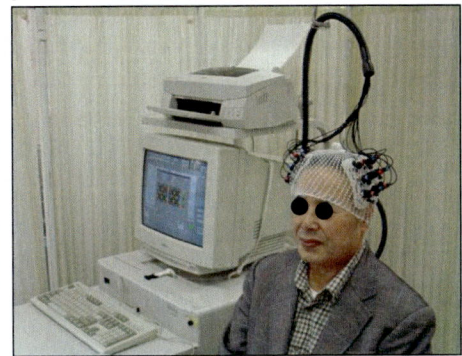

Figure 47. Optical Topography is composed of three parts. The light source generates a laser beam of 780nm and 830nm through optical fibers. The probe directs the modulated laser light onto the subject's head at the predetermined position and receives the reflection from the cranium. Reflected light goes to the avalanche photodiodes through the fibers. The third component is the controller, which converts optical signals into electrical signals. The controller analyses the data and displays the results. The probe consists of a soft plastic board on which the optical fibers are connected. The picture shows a pair of probe gears which measure both hemispheres simultaneously. The image represents the location of the probes of the optical topography attached to the bilateral temporal area.

All subjects were instructed to minimize head movements. Experimental tasks were clenching, gum chewing, mouth opening, tongue protrusion and phonation. During measurements, subjects alternated between 30 s of rest (off) and 10 s of tasks (on) for 5 times. The subjects were requested verbally to perform the task [226].

The cognition activation consisted of a 30 s pretask baseline, a 60 s word fluency task, and a 60 s posttask baseline in the word fluency task. The subjects were instructed to generate as many words whose initial syllables was /a/, /ka/, or /sa/ as they could. The three initial syllables changed in turn every 20 s during the 60 s task, to reduce the time during which the subjects were silent. The number of words generated during the fluency task was determined as a measure of task performance. The subjects were instructed to repeat the syllables /a/, /i/, /u/, /e/, and /o/ during the pretask and posttask baseline periods. The probes of the NIRS machine (Hitachi ETG-4000 Optical Topography, Hitachi Medical, Tokyo, Japan) were placed on a subject's frontal and bilateral temporal regions. The probes on the subject's frontal region measured the relative concentrations of Hb changes at 52 measurement points with the lowest probes positioned along the Fp1-Fp2 line, according to the international 10/20 system used in electroencephalography (Figure 48).

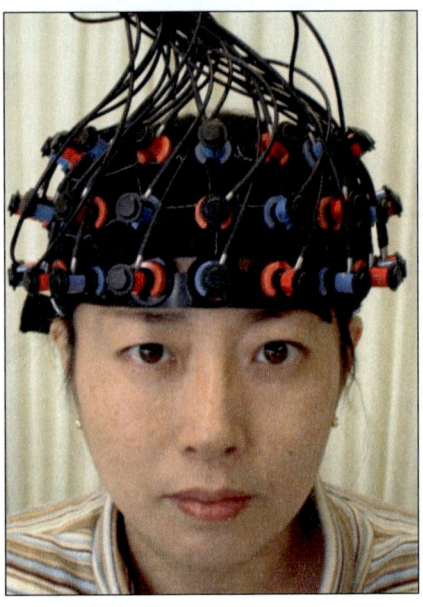

Figure 48. The position of the probes (Hitachi ETG-4000, 52 ch) for the measurement of the mean oxy-Hb, deoxy-Hb and total Hb. The probes on the subject's frontal region measured the relative concentrations of Hb changes at 52 measurement points with the lowest probes positioned along the Fp1-Fp2 line, according to the international 10/20 system used in electroencephalography.

The raw data from individual channels were digitally filtered at 0.02 Hz to remove long-time drift of baseline due to the artifacts. By averaging the time series over epochs, we obtained the hemodynamic response of each channel. The values of maximum minus minimum concentration of total-Hb during the tasks in each channel were calculated.

The event-related increase in Hb concentration was evident and all subjects showed significant changes over the bi-lateral temporal cortex that were consistent with the expected location of the masticatory cortex. In response to the tasks, distinctive increases in total-Hb, oxy-Hb and deoxy-Hb with high contrast were observed in the subjects. Figure 49 displays the typical measured mean signal changes of the task at 24 channels in the bi-lateral cortex of a subject [226]. Figure 50 presents a typical spatiotemporal hemodynamics over the cortex in response to the mouth opening and closing, tongue protrusion tasks [39]. The data revealed that the response to the test stimuli was vigorously detected as a localized increase in total-Hb concentration in the cortex. In contrast, no response was observed during sleep.

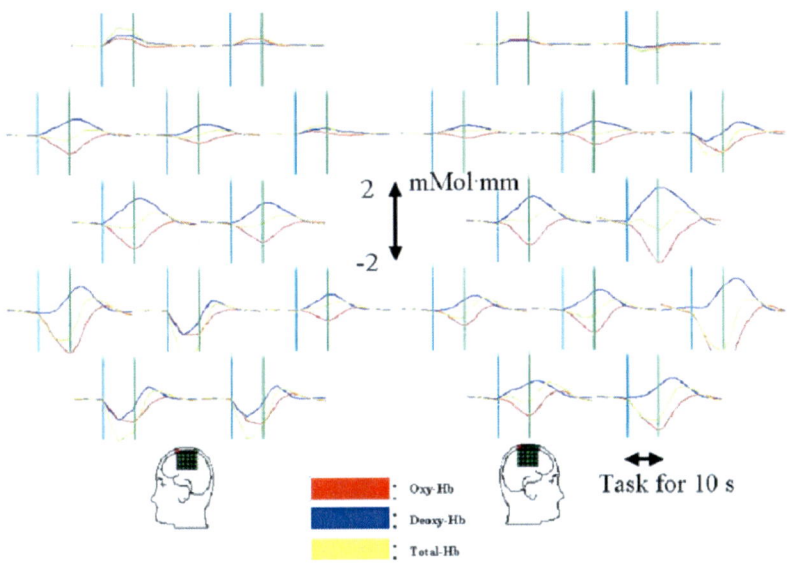

Figure 49. The plots show the average concentrations of the mean oxy-Hb (red), deoxy-Hb (blue) and total Hb (yellow) (mMol·mm) for successive 40 s windows of 5 times clenching tasks at 24 channels over the bilateral cortex of a subject. Left 12 channels indicate left lateral cortex. Light blue line points out the start of the clenching task and green line means the end of the task. The increase in Hb concentration is clear after starting of the task for consecutive 10 s windows.

In this study, the tasks significantly activated cerebral regional blood volume measured in the temporal cortex bi-laterally. In this study there were limitations, as the exact positions of the probes relative to the underlying brain were not clear. We thus focused on the variation of mean total Hb concentration in the measured area. Penfield and Boldrey [229] mapped the primary motor cortex in humans and demonstrated that the masticatory organs are represented in a comparatively large area on the inferior aspect of the primary motor cortex close to the lateral fissure. These regions are referred to as the masticatory center, although it is unclear why such a large cortex is devoted to the masticatory organ including teeth [230, 231]. Age related degeneration of somatosensory cortex occurs in humans and a strong relationship between mastication, learning and memory ability is suggested [232, 233]. Clinically, alterations in eating behavior are a major characteristic in the dementia population [234]. Moreover, a correlation was found between cerebral blood flow and neuropsychological outcome after injury, particularly in connection with verbal memory capacity, reasoning capacity and information processing speed [235].

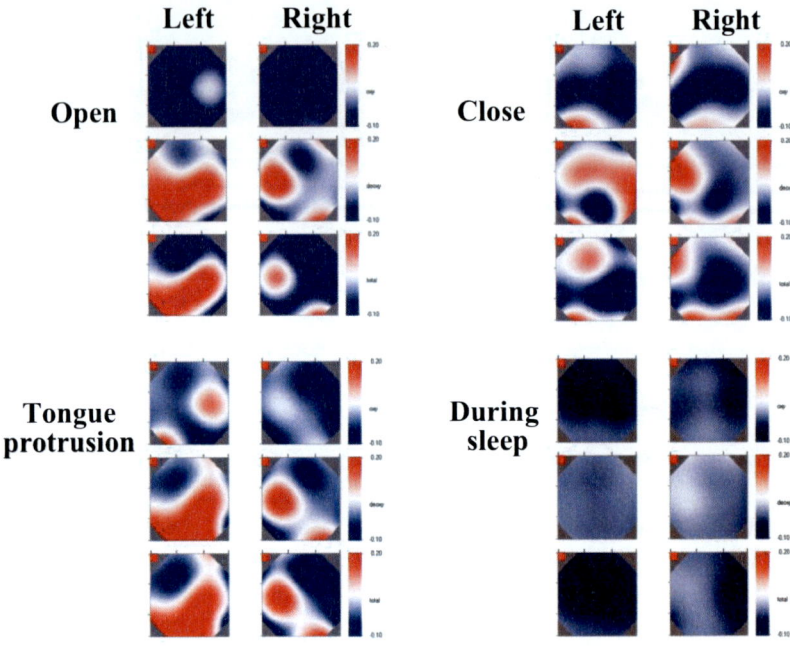

Figure 50. Pictures show typical spatiotemporal hemodynamics over the left temporal cortex of one participant in response to the maximum voluntary clenching task. Red areas denote increase in total Hb concentration. The series of images clearly demonstrate the response to the stimulation and the slow decay of the response over the lateral cortex particularly with prosthesis.

Because of disrupted sleep architecture and intermittent hypoxia during sleep, SAS leads to impaired daytime functioning in various neuropsychological and affective domains. These nocturnal respiratory disturbances cause daytime sleepiness and cognitive dysfunction. Deficits have been reported in attention and memory. Cognitive executive functions are associated with specific prefrontal-subcortical brain circuits. Therefore the executive control impairments have been suggested to be related to prefrontal lobe dysfunction due to intermittent nocturnal hypoxemia [236-238]. SAS can also have negative effects on mental process, behavior, and inter-personal relations. In a study [1], 24 % of SAS patients had seen psychiatrists for symptoms of depression and anxiety. 28 % of the patients had elevations on the depression scale and 36 % had elevations on the anxiety scale. Neuroimaging studies have revealed structural and functional brain abnormalities in psychiatric disorders. In a NIRS study, depression patients showed a smaller oxyhemoglobin increase in the prefrontal lobe during the first half of the word fluency task period [239].

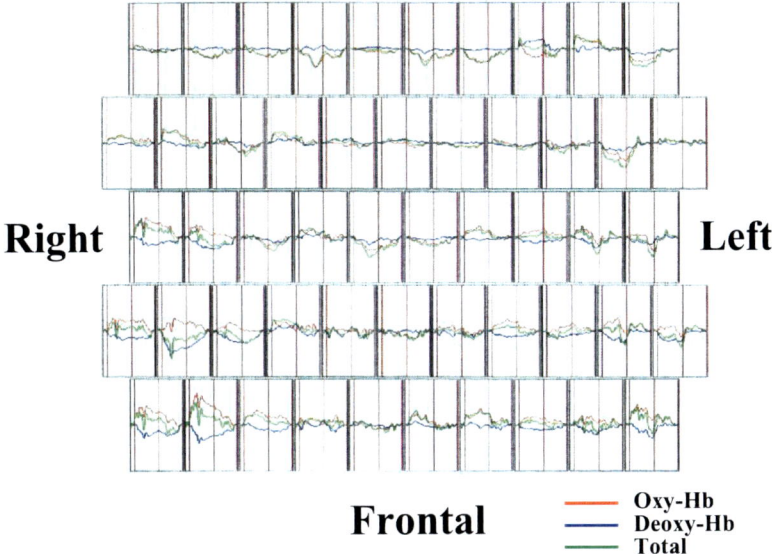

Figure 51. Waveforms of the mean oxy-Hb (red), deoxy-Hb (blue) and total Hb (yellow) (mMol·mm) concentration changes activated by the word fluency task in a patient with SAS.

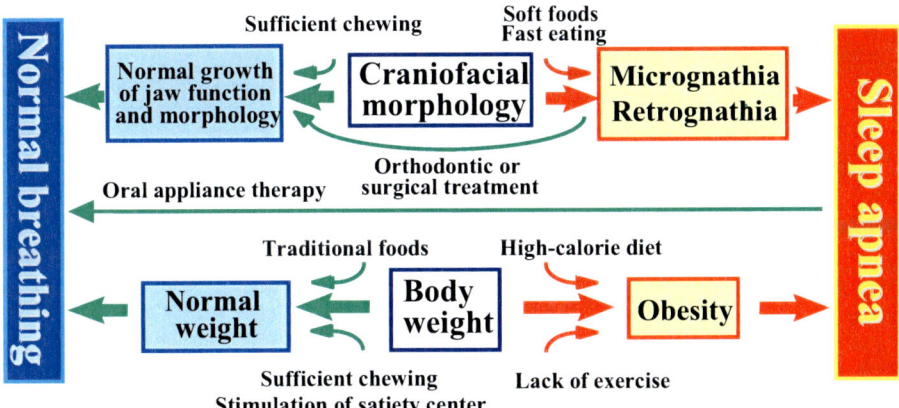

Figure 52. Craniofacial morphology and body weight are important factors for occurrence of SAS. Dental treatment is related to both factors. A custom to chew foods enough from the infancy and facilitate the growth development of a craniofacial structure, and dental

management including oral appliance therapy and maxillofacial surgical treatment to guide to both functionally and morphologically normal craniofacial morphology may prevent the patients from occurrence of SAS after reaching adulthood.

The oxyhemoglobin changes in the frontal lobe during the word fluency task have not been elucidated for SAS patients using NIRS. NIRS, with its noninvasiveness and high time resolution, can be a useful tool for research and clinical purposes in evaluating psychiatric aspects of SAS (Figure 51).

CONCLUSION

A combination of abnormal anatomy and physiology in the stomatognathic system is necessary to produce sleep-disordered breathing. Oral appliance therapy has a definite role in the treatment of sleep apnea and snoring. Enough chewing from childhood or orthodontic and other dental treatment can promote normal growth of craniofacial morphology, restrain overeating and obesity, and may prevent SAS (Figure 52). Dental approaches are very important in the treatment and prevention of SAS.

REFERENCES

[1] Guilleminault, C; Dement, WC. *Sleep apnea syndromes*. New York: Alan R. Liss; 1978.
[2] Wilms, D; Popovich, J; Conway, W; Fujita, S; Roth, T. Anatomic abnormalities in obstructive sleep apnea. *Ann. Otol. Rhinol. Laryngol.*, 1982; 91:595-596.
[3] Findley L, Unverzagt M, Suratt P: Automobile accidents involving patients with obstructive sleep apnea. *Am. Rev. Respir. Dis.*, 1988;138:337-340.
[4] Young, T; Palta, M; Dempsey, J; Skatrud, J; Weber, S; Badr S. The occurrence of sleep-disordered breathing among middle-aged adults. *N. Engl. J. Med.*, 1993;328:1230-1235.
[5] Brooks, D; Horner, RL; Kozar, LF; Render-Teixeira, CL; Phillipson, EA. Obstructive sleep apnea as a cause of systemic hypertension: evidence from a canine model. *J. Clin. Invest.*, 1997;99:106-109.
[6] Mooe, T; Rabben, T; Wiklund, U; Franklin, KA; Eriksson, P. Sleep-disordered breathing in men with coronary artery disease. *Chest*, 1996;109:659-663.
[7] Franklin, KA; Nilsson, JB; Sahlin, C; Näslund, U. Sleep apnoea and nocturnal angina. *Lancet*, 1995;345:1085-1086.
[8] Lugaresi, E; Cirignotta, F; Montagna, P. Pathogenic aspects of snoring and obstructive apnea syndrome. *Schweiz Med. Wschr*, 1988;118:1333-1337.
[9] Yoshida, K. Treatment and prognosis of sleep apnea syndrome. Oral appliance. *Mebio*, 2007;24:124-138.
[10] Kamijo, Y. *Oral anatomy*. Tokyo: Anatom; 1965.
[11] Harmon EM, Wynne JW, Black AJ: The effect of weight loss on sleep disordered breathing and oxygen desaturation in morbidly obese men. *Chest*, 1982;82:291-294.

[12] Cartwright, RD; Lloyd, S; Lilie, J; Krawitz, H. Sleep position training as treatment for sleep apnea syndrome: a preliminary study. *Sleep*, 1985;8:87-94.
[13] Meier-Ewert, K; Schäfer, H; Kloss, W. Treatment of sleep apnea by a mandibular protracting device. [Abstract]. Proceedings of the Seventh European Sleep Congress, Munich 1984;217.
[14] Kloss, W; Meier-Ewert, K; Schäfer, H. Zur Therapie des obstruktiven Schlaf-Apnoe-Syndroms. *Fortschr. Neurol. Psychiatr.*, 1986;54:267-271.
[15] Ichioka, M; Tojo, N; Yoshizawa, M; Chida, M; Miyazato, I; Taniai, S; Marumo, F; Nakagawa, K; Hasegawa, M. A dental device for the treatment of obstructive sleep apnea: a preliminary study. *Otolaryngol. Head Neck Surg.*, 1991;104:555-558.
[16] Schmidt-Nowara, WW; Mead, TE; Hays, MB. Treatment of snoring and obstructive sleep apnea with a dental orthosis. *Chest,* 1991;99:1378-1385.
[17] Nakazawa, Y; Sakamoto, T; Yasutake, R; Yamaga, K; Kotorii, T; Miyahara, Y; Ariyoshi, Y; Kameyama, T. Treatment of sleep apnea with prosthetic mandibular advancement (PMA). *Sleep*, 1992;15:499-504.
[18] Clark, GT; Arand, D; Chung, E; Tong, D. Effect of anterior mandibular positioning on obstructive sleep apnea. *Am. Rev. Respir. Dis.*, 1993; 147: 624-629.
[19] Yoshida, K. Prosthetic therapy for sleep apnea syndrome. *J. Prosthet. Dent*, 1994;72: 296-302.
[20] Marklund, M; Franklin, KA; Sahlin, C; Lundgren, R. The effect of a mandibular advancement device on apneas and sleep in patients with obstructive sleep apnea. *Chest*, 1998;113:707-713.
[21] Yoshida, K. Prothetische Therapie des Schlafapnoesyndroms: Wirksamkeit bei obstruktiven, gemischten und zentralen Apnoen. *Acta Med. Dent. Helv.*, 1998;3:75-78.
[22] Yoshida, K. Effects of a mandibular advancement device for the treatment of sleep apnea syndrome and snoring on respiratory function and sleep quality. *J. Craniomandibl. Pract.*, 2000;18:98-105.
[23] Sullivan, CE; Issa, FG; Berthon-Jones, M; Eves, L. Reversal of obstructive sleep apnoea by continuous positive airway pressure applied through the nares. *Lancet,* 1981;1:862–865.
[24] Kribbs, NB; Pack, AI; Kline, LR; Smith, PL; Schwartz, AR; Schubert, NM; Redline, S; Henry, JN; Getsy, JE; Dinges, DF. Objective measurement of patterns of nasal CPAP use by patients with obstructive sleep apnea. *Am. Rev. Respir. Dis.*, 1993;147:887-895.

[25] Naegele, B; Pepin, JL; Levy, P; Bonnet, C; Pellat, J; Feuerstein, C. Cognitive executive dysfunction in patients with obstructive sleep apnea syndrome (OSAS) after CPAP treatment. *Sleep*, 1998;21:392-397.
[26] Fujita, S; Conway, W; Zorick, F; Roth, T. Surgical correction of anatomic abnormalities in obstructive sleep apnea syndrome: Uvulopalatopharyngoplasty. *Otolaryngol. Head Neck Surg.*, 1981;89:923-934.
[27] Hochban, W; Brandenburg, U; Peter, JH. Surgical treatment of obstructive sleep apnea by maxillomandibular advancement. *Sleep*, 1994;17:624-629.
[28] Guilleminault, C; Simmons, FB; Motta, J; Cummiskey, J; Rosekind, M; Schroeder, JS; Dement, WC. Obstructive sleep apnea syndrome and tracheostomy: long-term follow-up experience. *Arch. Intern. Med.*, 1981;141:985-988.
[29] Schmidt-Nowara, W; Lowe, A; Wiegand, L; Cartwright, R; Perez-Guerra, F; Menn, S. Oral appliances for the treatment of snoring and obstructive sleep apnea: a review. *Sleep*, 1995;18:501-510.
[30] Ferguson, KA; Lowe, AA. Oral appliances for sleep-disordered breathing. In: Kryger MH, Roth T, Dement WC, editors. *Principles and practice of sleep medicine*. Fourth edition. Philadelphia: Elsevier Saunders; 2005:1098-1108.
[31] Ferguson, KA; Cartwright, R; Rogers, R; Schmidt-Nowara, W. Oral appliances for snoring and obstructive sleep apnea: a review. *Sleep*, 2006;29:244-262.
[32] Hoffstein, V. Review of oral appliances for treatment of sleep-disordered breathing. *Sleep Breath.*, 2007;11:1-22.
[33] American Sleep Disorders Association Standards of Practice Committee. Practice parameters for the treatment of snoring and obstructive sleep apnea with oral appliances. *Sleep*, 1995;18:511-513.
[34] Ferguson, KA; Ono, T; Lowe, AA; Keenan, SP; Fleetham, JA. A randomized crossover study of an oral appliance vs nasal-continuous positive airway pressure in the treatment of mild-moderate obstructive sleep apnea. *Chest*, 1996;109:1269-1275.
[35] Clark, GT; Blumenfeld, I; Yoffe, N; Peled, E; Lavie, P. A crossover study comparing the efficacy of continuous positive airway pressure with anterior mandibular positioning devices on patients with obstructive sleep apnea. *Chest*, 1996;109:1477-1483.
[36] Miljeteig, H; Mateika, S; Haight, JS; Cole, P; Hoffstein, V. Subjective and objective assessment of uvulopalatopharyngoplasty for treatment of snoring and obstructive sleep apnea. *Am. J. Resp. Crit. Care Med.*, 1994;150:1286-1290.

[37] Riley, RW; Powell, NB; Guilleminault, C. Obstructive sleep apnea syndrome: a review of 306 a review of 306 consecutively treated surgical patients. *Otolaryngeal. Head Neck Surg.,* 1993;108:117-125..
[38] Mylonas, T; Yoshida, K; Siebert, GK. Apnoe-Schiene für Patienten mit Schlaf-Apnoe-Syndrom. *Zahnärztl. Welt.,* 1994;103:432-434.
[39] Yoshida, K. Effect of oral appliance. Shiomi T, Kikuchi M, editors. *Clinical sleep medicine and dentistry.* Tokyo: Hyoron Publishers; 2004:150-157.
[40] Yoshida, K. Elastic retracted oral appliance to treat sleep apnea in mentally impaired patients and patients with neuromuscular disabilities. *J. Prosthet. Dent.,* 1999;81:196-201.
[41] Lowe, AA. Dental appliances for the treatment of snoring and/or obstructive sleep apnea. In: Kryger MH, Roth T, Dement W, editors. *Principles and practice of sleep medicine.* Second edition. Philadelphia: WB Saunders; 1994:722-35.
[42] Cartwright, RD; Samelson, CF. The effects of a nonsurgical treatment for obstructive sleep apnea. The tongue-retaining device. *JAMA,* 1982;248:705-709.
[43] Rose,E; Staats, R; Virchow, C; Jonas, IE. A comparative study of two mandibular advancement appliances for the treatment of obstructive sleep apnoea. *Eur. J. Orthod.,* 2002;24:191-198.
[44] Yoshida, K. Oral device therapy for the upper airway resistance syndrome patient. *J. Prosthet. Dent.,* 2002;87:427-430.
[45] Guilleminault, C; Stoohs, R; Clerk, A; Cetel, M; Maistros, P. A cause of excessive daytime sleepiness: the upper airway resistance syndrome. *Chest,* 1993;104:781-787.
[46] Guilleminault, C; Stoohs, R; Kim, Y; Chervin, R; Black, J; Clerk, A. Upper airway sleep-disordered breathing in women. *Ann. Intern. Med.,* 1995;122:493-501.
[47] Exar, E. N; Collop, N. A. The upper airway resistance syndrome. *Chest,* 1999;115:1127-1139.
[48] Isono, S; Tanaka, A; Sho, Y; Konno, A; Nishino, T. Advancement of the mandible improves velopharyngeal airway patency. *J. Appl. Physiol.,* 1995;79:2132-2138.
[49] Ishida, M; Inoue, Y; Suto, Y; Okamoto, K; Ryoke, K; Higami, S; Suzuki, T; Kawahara, R. Mechanism of action and therapeutic indication of prosthetic mandibular advancement in obstructive sleep apnea syndrome. *Psychiatry Clin. Neurosci.,* 1998;52:227-229.

[50] Eveloff, SE; Rosenberg, CL; Carlisle, CC; Millman, RP. Efficacy of a Herbst mandibular advancement device in obstructive sleep apnea. *Am. J. Respir. Crit. Care Med.*, 1994;149:905-909.

[51] Mayer, G; Meier-Ewert, K. Cephalometric predictors for orthopaedic mandibular advancement in obstructive sleep apnoea. *Eur. J. Orthod.*, 1995;17:35-43.

[52] Johal, A; Battagel, JM. An investigation into the changes in airway dimension and the efficacy of mandibular advancement appliances in subjects with obstructive sleep apnoea. *Br. J. Orthod.*, 1999;26:205-210.

[53] Battagel, JM; Johal, A; L'Estrange, PR; Croft, CB; Kotecha, B. Changes in airway and hyoid position in response to mandibular protrusion in subjects with obstructive sleep apnoea (OSA). *Eur. J. Orthod.*, 1999;21:363-376.

[54] Liu, Y; Park, YC, Lowe, AA; Fleetham, JA. Supine cephalometric analyses of an adjustable oral appliance used in the treatment of obstructive sleep apnea. *Sleep Breath.*, 2000;4:59-66.

[55] Gao, XM; Zeng, XL; Fu, MK; Huang, XZ. Magnetic resonance imaging of the upper airway in obstructive sleep apnea before and after oral appliance therapy. *Chin. J. Dent. Res.*, 1999;2:27-35.

[56] Gale, DJ; Sawyer, RH; Woodcock, A; Stone, P; Thompson, R; O'Brien, K. Do oral appliances enlarge the airway in patients with obstructive sleep apnoea? A prospective computerized tomographic study. *Eur. J. Orthod.*, 200;22:159-168.

[57] Cobo, J, Canut, JA; Carlos, F; Vijande, M; Llamas, JM. Changes in the upper airway of patients who wear a modified functional appliance to treat obstructive sleep apnea. *Int. J. Adult Orthod Orthognath Surg.*, 1995;10:53-57.

[58] Ryan, CF; Love, LL; Peat, D; Fleetham, JA; Lowe, AA. Mandibular advancement oral appliance therapy for obstructive sleep apnoea: effect on awake calibre of the velopharynx. *Thorax,* 1999:54:972-977.

[59] Yoshida, K. Effect of a prosthetic appliance for sleep apnea syndrome on masticatory and tongue muscle activity. *J. Prosthet. Dent.*, 1998;79:537-544.

[60] Tsuiki, S; Ono, T; Kuroda, T. Mandibular advancement modulates respiratory-related genioglossus electromyographic activity. *Sleep Breath.*, 2000;4:53-54.

[61] Mehta, A; Qian, J; Petocz, P; Darendeliler, MA; Cistulli PA. A randomized, controlled study of a mandibular advancement splint for obstructive sleep apnea. *Am. J. Respir. Crit. Care Med.*, 2001;163:1457-1461.

[62] Gotsopoulos, H; Chen, C; Qian, J; Cistulli PA. Oral appliance therapy improves symptoms in obstructive sleep apnea: a randomized, controlled trial. *Am. J. Respir. Crit. Care Med.*, 2002;166:743-748.

[63] Ng, AT; Gotsopoulos, H; Qian, J; Cistulli, PA. Effect of oral appliance therapy on upper airway collapsibility in obstructive sleep apnea. *Am. J. Respir. Crit. Care Med.*, 2003;168:238-241.

[64] Rechtschaffen, A; Kales, A. A manual of standardized terminology, techniques and scoring system for sleep states of human subjects. NIH publication number 204, Washington: U.S. Government Printing Office, 1968.

[65] O'Sullivan, RA; Hillman, DR; Mateljan, R; Pantin, C; Finucane, KE. Mandibular advancement splint: an appliance to treat snoring and obstructive sleep apnea. *Am. J. Respir. Crit. Care Med.*, 1995;151:194-198.

[66] Yoshida, K. Effect on blood pressure of oral appliance therapy for sleep apnea syndrome. *Int. J. Prosthodont.*, 2006:19;61-66.

[67] Carskadon, MA; Dement, WC. Normal human sleep: an overview. In: Kryger MH, Roth T, Dement WC, editors, Principles and practice of sleep medicine, Second edition. Philadelphia: WB Saunders, 1994;16-25.

[68] Giles, TL; Lasserson, TJ; Smith, BJ; White, J; Wright, J; Cates, CJ. Continuous positive airways pressure for obstructive sleep apnoea in adults. *Cochrane Database Syst. Rev.*, 2006.

[69] Grote, L; Ploch, T; Heitmann, J; Knaack, L; Penzel, T; Peter, JH. Sleep-related breathing disorder is an independent risk factor for systemic hypertension. *Am. J. Respir. Crit. Care Med.*, 1999;160:1875-1882.

[70] Peppard, PE; Young, T; Palta, M; Skatrud, J. Prospective study of the association between sleep-disordered breathing and hypertension. *N. Engl. J. Med.*, 2000;342:1378–1384.

[71] Jennum, P; Wildschiodtz, G; Christensen, NJ; Schwartz, T. Blood pressure, catecholamines, and pancreatic polypeptide in obstructive sleep apnea with and without nasal continuous positive airway pressure (nCPAP) treatment. *Am. J. Hypertens.*, 1989 2:847-852.

[72] Wilcox, I; Grunstein, RR; Hedner, JA; Doyle, J; Collins, FL; Fletcher, PJ; Kelly, DT; Sullivan, CE. Effect of nasal continuous positive airway pressure during sleep on 24-hour blood pressure in obstructive sleep apnea. *Sleep*, 1993;16:539-544.

[73] Voogel, AJ, van Steenwijk, RP; Karemaker, JM; van Montfrans, GA. Effects of treatment of obstructive sleep apnea on circadian hemodynamics. *J. Auton Nerv. Syst.*, 1999;77:179-183.

[74] Engleman, HM; Gough, K; Martin, SE; Kingshott, RN; Padfield, PL; Douglas, NJ. Ambulatory blood pressure on and off continuous positive airway pressure therapy for the sleep apnea/hypopnea syndrome: effects in "non-dippers". *Sleep*, 1996;19:378-381.

[75] Dimsdale, JE; Loredo, JS; Profant, J. Effect of continuous positive airway pressure on blood pressure: a placebo trial. *Hypertension*, 2000;35:144-147.

[76] Barnes, M; McEvoy, RD; Banks, S; Tarquinio, N; Murray, CG; Vowles, N; Pierce, RJ. Efficacy of positive airway pressure and oral appliance in mild to moderate obstructive sleep apnea. *Am. J. Respir. Crit. Care Med.*, 2004; 170:656-664.

[77] Faccenda, JF; Mackay, TW; Boon, NA; Douglas, NJ. Randomized placebo-controlled trial of continuous positive airway pressure on blood pressure in the sleep apnea-hypopnea syndrome. *Am. J. Respir. Crit. Care Med.*, 2001; 163:344-348.

[78] Pepperell, JC; Ramdassingh-Dow, S; Crosthwaite, N; Mullins, R; Jenkinson, C; Stradling, JR; Davies RJ. Ambulatory blood pressure after therapeutic and subtherapeutic nasal continuous positive airway pressure for obstructive sleep apnoea: a randomized parallel trial. *Lancet*, 2002;359:204-210.

[79] Becker, HF; Jerrentrup, A; Ploch, T; Grote, L; Penzel, T; Sullivan, CE, Becker, JH. Effect of nasal continuous positive airway pressure treatment on blood pressure in patients with obstructive sleep apnea. *Circulation*, 2003;107:68-73.

[80] Gotsopoulos, H; Kelly, JJ; Cistulli, PA. Oral appliance therapy reduces blood pressure in obstructive sleep apnea: a randomized, controlled trial. *Sleep*, 2004;27:934-941.

[81] Lam, B; Sam, K; Mok, WY; Cheung, MT; Fong, DY; Lam, JC; Lam, DC; Yam, LY; Ip, MS. Randomised study of three non-surgical treatments in mild to moderate obstructive sleep apnoea. *Thorax*, 2007;62:354-359.

[82] MacMahon, S; Peto, R; Cutler, J; Collins, R; Sorlie, P; Neaton, J; Abbott, R; Godwin, J; Dyer, A; Stamler, J. Blood pressure, stroke, and coronary heart disease. Part 1, prolonged differences in blood pressure: prospective observational studies corrected for the regression dilution bias. *Lancet*, 1990;335:765-774.

[83] Cohen, MC; Rohtla, KM; Lavery, CE; Muller, JE; Mittleman, MA. Meta-analysis of the morning excess of acute myocardial infarction and sudden cardiac death. *Am. Heart J.*, 1997;79:1512-1515.

[84] Elliot, WJ. Circadian variation in the timing of stroke onset: a meta-analysis. *Stroke*, 1998;29:992-996.

[85] Carlson, JT; Hedner, J; Elam, M; Ejnell, H; Sellgren, J; Wallin, BG. Augmented resting sympathetic activity in awake patients with obstructive sleep apnea. *Chest,* 1993;103:1763-1768.
[86] Hla, KM; Young, TB; Bidwell, T; Palta, M; Skatrud, JB; Dempsy, J. Sleep apnea and hypertension: a population-based study. *Ann. Intern. Med.,* 1994;120:382-388.
[87] Millman, RP; Redline, S; Carlisle, CC; Assaf, AR; Levinson, PD. Daytime hypertension in obstructive sleep apnoea: prevalence and contributing factors. *Chest,* 1991;99:861-866.
[88] Otsuka, R; Ribeiro de Almeida, F; Lowe, AA; Linden, W; Ryan, F. The effect of oral appliance therapy on blood pressure in patients with obstructive sleep apnea. *Sleep Breath.,* 2006;10:29-36.
[89] Yoshida, K. A polysomnographic study on influence of masticatory and tongue muscle activity in occurrence of sleep apnea. *J. Oral Rehabil.,* 1998;25:603-609.
[90] Johns, MW. A new method for measuring daytime sleepiness, the Epworth sleepiness scale. *Sleep,* 1991;14:540-545.
[91] Carskadon, MA; Dement, WC; Mitler, MM; Roth, T; Westbrook, PR; Keenan, S. Guidelines for the multiple sleep latency test (MSLT): a standard measure of sleepiness. *Sleep,* 1986;9:519-524.
[92] Loube, DI; Andrada, TF. Comparison of respiratory polysomnographic parameters in matched cohorts of upper airway resistance and obstructive sleep apnea syndrome patients. *Chest,* 1999;115:1519-1524.
[93] Bahammam, AS; Tate, R; Manfreda, J; Kryger, MH. Upper airway resistance syndrome: effect of nasal dilation, sleep stage, and sleep position. *Sleep,* 1999;22:592-598.
[94] Almeida, FR; Lowe, AA; Sung, JO; Tsuiki, S; Otsuka, R. Long-term sequellae of oral appliance therapy in obstructive sleep apnea patients: Part 1. Cephalometric analysis. *Am. J. Orthod. Dentofacial Orthop.,* 2006; 129:195-204.
[95] Almeida, FR; Lowe, AA; Otsuka, R; Fastlicht, S; Farbood, M; Tsuiki, S. Long-term sequellae of oral appliance therapy in obstructive sleep apnea patients: Part 2. Study-model analysis. *Am. J. Orthod. Dentofacial Orthop.,* 2006;129:205-213.
[96] Harper, R; Sauerland, EK. The role of the tongue in sleep apnea. In: Guilleminault C, Dement WC, editors, *Sleep apnea syndromes,* New York: Alan R. Liss; 1978:219-234.
[97] Yoshida, K. Influence of sleep posture on response to oral appliance therapy for sleep apnea syndrome. *Sleep,* 2001;24:538-544.

[98] Remmers, JE; deGroot, WJ; Sauerland, EK; Anch, AM. Pathogenesis of upper airway occlusion during sleep. *J. Appl. Physiol.*, 1978;44:931-938.

[99] Yoshida, K. Kau- und Zungenmuskelaktivität während des Schlafens bei Patienten mit Schlafapnoesyndrom. In: Struppler A, editor, *Motodiagnostik-Mototherapie II*, Jena: Jena University Press; 1994:161-164.

[100] Kovacenic-Ristanovic, R; Alger, G; Cartwright, R. Cephalometric analysis in positional sleep apneics. *Sleep Res.*, 1989;18:249.

[101] Dwyer, T; Ponsoby, ALB; Newman, NM; Gibbons, LE. Prospective cohort study of prone sleeping position and sudden infant death syndrome. *Lancet*, 1991;337:1244-1247.

[102] Tonkin, S. Sudden infant death syndrome: hypothesis of causation. *Pediatrics*, 1975;55:650-661.

[103] Tonkin, SL; Partridge, J. The pharyngeal effect of partial nasal obstruction. *Pediatrics*, 1979;63:261-271.

[104] Hillarp, B; Nylander, G; Rosén, I; Wickström, O. Videoradiography of patients with habitual snoring and/or sleep apnea. *Acta Radiol.*, 1996;37:307-314.

[105] Cartwright, R. Effect of sleep position on sleep apnea severity. *Sleep*, 1984;7:110-114.

[106] Kavey, NB; Blitzer, A; Gidro-Frank, S; Korstanje, K. Sleeping position and sleep apnea syndrome. *Am. J. Otolaryngol.*, 1985;6:373-377.

[107] George, CF; Millar, TW; Kryger, MH. Sleep apnea and body position during sleep. *Sleep*, 1988;11:90-99.

[108] Grote, L; Hedner, J; Grunstein, R; Kraiczi, H. Therapy with nCPAP: incomplete elimination of sleep related breathing disorder. *Eur. Respir. J.*, 2000;16:921-927.

[109] Thumm, J; Siebert, GK; Mylonas, T; Yoshida, K; Meier-Ewert, K. Langzeitakzeptanz von Esmarch-Schiene bei Patienten mit obstruktiven Schlaf-Apnoe-Syndrom. *Zahnärztl. Welt.*, 1995;104:458-462.

[110] Report of the American Sleep Disorders Association. Practice parameters for the treatment of snoring and obstructive sleep apnea in adults: the efficacy of surgical modifications of the upper airway. *Sleep*, 1996;19:152-155.

[111] Powell, NB; Riley, RW; Guilleminault, C. Surgical management of sleep-disordered breathing. In: Kryger MH, Roth T, Dement WC, editors. *Principles and practice of sleep medicine*. Fourth edition. Philadelphia: Elsevier Saunders; 2005;1081-1097.

[112] Prinsell, JR. Maxillomandibular advancement surgery in a site-specific treatment approach for obstructive sleep apnea in 50 consecutive patients. *Chest*, 1999;116:1519-1529.
[113] Nishida, M; Iizuka, T; Murakami, K; Kawamura, K; Hyo, Y; Ono, T. Surgical correction of severe retrognathia associated with respiratory distress in an adult patient: report of a case. *Jpn. J. Jaw Deform.*, 1986;5:22-24.
[114] Hochban, W; Conradt, R; Brandenburg, U; Heitmann, J; Peter, JH. Surgical maxillofacial treatment of obstructive sleep apnea. *Plast. Reconstr. Surg.*, 1997;99:619-626.
[115] Bettega, G; Pepin, JL; Veale, D; Deschaux, C; Raphael, B; Levy, P. Obstructive sleep apnea syndrome. Fifty-one consecutive patients treated by maxillofacial surgery. *Am. J. Respir. Crit. Care Med.*, 2000;162:641-649.
[116] Prinsell, J. R. Maxillomandibular advancement surgery for obstructive sleep apnea syndrome. *J. Am. Dent. Assoc.*, 2002;133:1489-1497.
[117] Waite, PD; Wooten, V; Lachner, J; Guyette, RF. Maxillomandibular advancement surgery in 23 patients with obstructive sleep apnea syndrome. *J. Oral Maxillofac. Surg.*, 1989;47:1256-1261.
[118] Obwegeser, H. The indication for surgical correction of mandibular deformity by the sagittal splitting technique. *Brit. J. Oral Surg.*, 1964;1:157-171.
[119] Moore, MH; Guzman-Stein, G; Proudman, TW; Abbott, AH; Netherway, DJ. Mandibular lengthening by distraction for airway obstruction in Treacher-Collins syndrome. *J. Craniofac. Surg.*, 1994;5:22-25.
[120] Cohen, SR; Simms, C; Burstein, FD. Mandibular distraction osteogenesis in the treatment of upper airway obstruction in children with craniofacial deformities. *Plast. Reconstr. Surg.*, 1998;101:312-318.
[121] Li, KK; Powell, NB; Riley, RW; Guilleminault, C. Distraction osteogenesis in adult obstructive sleep apnea surgery: a preliminary report. *J. Oral Maxillofac. Surg.*, 2002;60:6-10.
[122] Shimizu, I; Takahashi, K; Murakami, K; Yokoe, Y; Iizuka, T. Retromandible with temporomandibular joint disorders treated by distraction osteogenesis to prevent progressive condylar resorption - a case report -. *Jpn. J. Jaw Deform.*, 2004;14:75-82.
[123] Lindeh, J. Karring T, Lang NP, editors. *Clinical periodontology and implant dentistry*. Munksgaard: Blackwell; 2005.
[124] Yoshida, K. Oral hygiene and sleep. The Japanese Society of Sleep Research, editor. *Sleep medicine*, Tokyo: Asakura Shoten; 2009;644-648.

[125] Saito, T; Shimazaki, Y; Sakamoto, M. Obesity and periodontitis. *N. Engl. J. Med.*, 339: 482-483, 1997.
[126] Iwamoto, Y; Nishimura, F; Nakagawa, M; Sugimoto, H; Shikata, K; Makino, H; Fukuda, T; Tsuji, T; Iwamoto, M; Murayama, Y. The effect of antimicrobial treatment on circulating tumor necrosis factor-alpha and glycated hemoglobin level in patients with type 2 diabetes. *J. Periodontol.*, 2001;72:774-778.
[127] Uysal, KT; Wiesbrock, SM; Marino, MW; Hotamisligil, GS. Protection from obesity-induced insulin resistance in mice lacking TNF-alpha function. *Nature*, 1997;389:610-614.
[128] Rattazzi, M; Puato, M; Faggin, E; Bertipaglia, B; Zambon, A; Pauletto, P. C-reactive protein and interleukin-6 in vascular disease: culprits or passive bystanders? *J. Hypertens.*, 2003;21:1787-1803.
[129] Lakka, HM; Laaksonen, DE; Lakka, TA; Niskanen, LK; Kumpusalo, E; Tuomilehto, J; Salonen, JT. The metabolic syndrome and total and cardiovascular disease mortality in middle-aged men. *JAMA*, 2002; 288:2709-2716.
[130] Yoshida, K; Kaji, R; Hamano, T; Kohara, N; Kimura, J; Shibasaki, H; Iizuka, T. Cortical potentials associated with voluntary mandibular movements. *J. Dent. Res.*, 2000;79:1514-1518.
[131] Yoshida, K; Iizuka, T. Contingent negative variation for voluntary mandibular movements in humans. *J. Oral. Rehabil.*, 2005:32;871-879.
[132] Yoshida, K; Maezawa, H; Nagamine, T; Fukuyama, H; Murakami, K; Iizuka, T. Somatosensory evoked magnetic fields to air-puff stimulation on the soft palate. *Neurosci. Res.*, 2006:55;116-122.
[133] Larson, CR; Byrd, KE; Garthewaite, CR; Luschei, ES. Alterations in the pattern of mastication after ablations of the lateral precentral cortex in rhesus macaques. *Exp. Neurol.*, 1980;70:638-651.
[134] Lund, JP; Lamarre, Y. Activity of neurons in the lower precentral cortex during voluntary and rhythmical jaw movements in the monkey. *Exp. Brain Res.*, 1974;19:282-299.
[135] Hoffman, DS; Luschei, ES. Responses of monkey precentral cortical cells during a controlled jaw bite task. *J. Neurophysiol.*, 1980;44:333-348.
[136] Hollowell, DE; Suratt, PM. Mandible position and activation of submental and masseter muscles during sleep. *J. Appl. Physiol.*, 1991;71:2267-2273.
[137] Sauerland, EK; Sauerland, BAT; Orr, WC; Harrison, LE. Non-invasive electromyography of human genioglossal (tongue) activity. *Electromyogr. Clin. Neurophysiol.*, 1981;21:279-286.

[138] Morikawa, S; Safar, P; Decarlo, J. Influence of the head-jaw position upon upper airway patency. *Anesthesiology*, 1961;22:265-270.
[139] White, DP. Central sleep apnea. *Med. Clin. North Am.*, 1985;69:1205-1219.
[140] Önal, E; Lopata, M; O'Connor, TD. Poathogenesis of apneas in hypersomnia-sleep apnea syndrome. *Am. Rev. Respir. Dis.*, 1982;125:167-174.
[141] Kornhuber, HH; Deecke, L. Hirnpotentialänderungen bei Wirkürbewegungen und passiven Bewegungen des Menschen: Bereitschaftpotential und reafferente Potentiale. *Pflügers Arch. Ges. Physiol.*, 1965;284:1-17.
[142] Shibasaki, H; Barrett, G; Halliday, E; Halliday, AM. Components of the movement-related cortical potential and their scalp topography. *Electroencephalogr. Clin. Neurophysiol.*, 1980;49:213-226.
[143] Ikeda, A; Shibasaki, H. Invasive recording of movement-related cortical potentials in humans. *J. Clin. Neurophysiol.*, 1992;9:509-520.
[144] Shibasaki, H. Movement-related cortical potentials. In: Halliday AM. editor. *Evoked potentials in clinical testing.* Second edition. Edinburgh: Churchill Livingston; 1993;523-537.
[145] Nakajima, I; Tanaka, Y; Uchida, A; Sakai, T; Akasaka, M; Mori, A; Sumino, R. Cortical potentials associated with voluntary movement in humans. *Neurosci. Res.,* 1991;10:285-289.
[146] Wohlert, AB. Event-related brain potentials preceding speech and nonspeech oral movements of varying complexity. *J. Speech Hear Res.*, 1993;36:897-905.
[147] Ikeda, A; Lüders, HO; Burgess, RC; Sakamoto, A; Klem, GH; Morris, HH; Shibasaki, H. Generator locations of movement-related potentials with tongue protrusion and vocalizations: subdural recording in human. *Electroencephalogr. Clin. Neurophysiol.*, 1995;96:310-328.
[148] Oldfield, RC. The assessment and analysis of handedness: the Edingburgh inventory. *Neuropsychologia*, 1971;9:97-113.
[149] Yoshida, K. An electromyographic study on the superior head of the lateral pterygoid muscle during mastication from the standpoint of condylar movement. *J. Jpn. Prosthodont. Soc.*, 1992;36:340-350.
[150] Yoshida, K. Eigenschaften der Kaumuskelaktivität während verschiedener Unterkieferbewegungen bei Patienten mit Diskusverlagerungen ohne Reposition. *Stomatologie*, 1999;96:107-121.
[151] Christensen, LV; Radue, JT. Lateral preference in mastication: a feasibility study. *J. Oral Rehabil.* 1985;12:421-427.

[152] Barrett, G; Shibasaki, H; Neshige, R. A computer-assisted method for averaging movement-related cortical potentials with respect to EMG onset. *Electroencephalogr. Clin. Neurophysiol.*, 1985;60:276-281.
[153] Grözinger, B; Kornhuber, H. H; Kriebel, J. Human cerebral potentials preceding speech production, phonation, and movements of the mouth and tongue, with reference to respiratory and extracerebral potentials. In: Desmedt JE, editor. *Language and hemispheric specialization in man: cerebral ERPs*. Progress in clinical neurophysiology, Vol. 3, Basel: Karger; 1977;87-103.
[154] Brooker, BH; Donald, MW. Contribution of the speech musculature to apparent human EEG asymmetries prior to vocalization. *Brain Lang.*, 1980;9:226-245.
[155] Deecke, L; Engel, M; Lang, W; Kornhuber, HH. Bereitschaftspotentials preceding speech after breath holding. *Exp. Brain Res.*, 1986;65:219-223.
[156] Neshige, R; Lüders, H; Shibasaki, H. Recording of movement-related potentials from scalp and cortex in man. *Brain,* 1988;111:719-736.
[157] Shibasaki, H; Barrett, G; Halliday, E; Halliday, AM. Cortical potentials associated with voluntary foot movement in man. *Electroencephalogr. Clin. Neurophysiol.*, 1981;49:213-226.
[158] Kitamura, J; Shibasaki, H; Kondo, T. A cortical slow potential is larger before an isolated movement of a single finger than simultaneous movement of two fingers. *Electroencephalogr. Clin. Neurophysiol.*, 1993;86:252-258.
[159] Benecke, R; Dick, JPR; Rothwell, JC; Day, BL; Marsden, CD. Increase of the Bereitschaftpotential in simultaneous and sequential movements. *Electroencephalogr. Clin. Neurophysiol.*, 1985;62:347-352.
[160] Simonetta, M; Clanet, M; Rascol, O. Bereitschaftspotentials in a simple movement or in a motor sequence starting with the same simple movement. *Electroencephalogr. Clin. Neurophysiol.*, 1991;81:129-134.
[161] Kristeva, R. Bereitschaftspotential of pianists. *Ann. N. Y. Acad. Sci.,* 1984;425:477-482.
[162] Walter, WG; Cooper, R; Aldridge, VJ; McCallum, WC; Winter, AL. Contingent negative variation: an electric sign of sensorimotor association and expectancy in the human brain. *Nature,* 1964;203:380-384.
[163] Brunia, CH. Movement and stimulus preceding negativity. *Biol. Psychol.*, 1988;26:165-178.
[164] Rosahl, SK; Knight, RT. Role of prefrontal cortex in generation of the CNV. *Cereb. Cortex*, 1995;2:123-134.
[165] Gaillard, AW. Effects of warning signal modality on the contingent negative variation (CNV). *Biol. Psychol.*, 1976;4:139-154.

[166] Rohrbaugh, JW; Syndulko, K; Lindsley, DB. Cortical slow negative waves following non-paired stimuli: effects of modality, intensity and rate of stimulation. *Electroencephalogr. Clin. Neurophysiol.*, 1979;46:416-427.

[167] Brunia, CHM; Damen, EJP. Distribution of slow brain potentials related to motor preparation and stimulus anticipation in a time estimation task. *Electroencephalogr. Clin. Neurophysiol.*, 1988;69:234-243.

[168] Verleger, R; Wauschkuhn, B; Van der Lubbe, RHJ; Jaskowski, P; Trillenberg, P. Posterior and anterior contributions of hand-movement preparation to late CNV. *J. Psychophysiol.*, 2000;14:69-86.

[169] Ikeda, A; Lüders, HO; Collura, TF; Burgess, RC; Morris, HH; Hamano, T; Shibasaki H. Subdural potentials at orbitofrontal and mesial prefrontal areas accompanying anticipation and decision making in humans: a comparison with Bereitschaftspotential. *Electroencephalogr. Clin. Neurophysiol.*, 1996;98:206-212.

[170] Ikeda, A; Shibasaki, H; Kaji, R; Terada, K; Nagamine, T; Honda, M; Kimura J. Dissociation between contingent negative variation (CNV) and Bereitschaftspotential (BP) in patients with parkinsonism. *Electroencephalogr. Clin. Neurophysiol.*, 1997;102:142-151.

[171] Kaji, R; Ikeda, A; Ikeda, T; Kubori, T; Mezaki, T; Kohara, N; Kanda, M; Nagamine, T; Honda, M; Rothwell, JC; Kimura, J. Physiological study of cervical dystonia: Task-specific abnormality in contingent negative variation. *Brain*, 1995;118:511-522.

[172] Hamano, T; Kaji, R; Katayama, M; Kubori, T; Ikeda, A; Shibasaki, H; Kimura, J. Abnormal contingent negative variation in writer's cramp. *Electroencephalogr. Clin. Neurophysiol.*, 1999;110:508-515.

[173] Deuschl, G; Toro, C; Matsumoto, J; Hallett, M. Movement-related cortical potentials in writer's cramp. *Ann. Neurol.*, 1995;38:862-868.

[174] Van der Kamp, W; Rothwell, JC; Thompson, PD; Day, BL; Marsden, CD. The movement-related cortical potential is abnormal in patients with idiopathic torsion dystonia. *Mov. Disord.*, 1995;10:630-633.

[175] Yoshida, K; Kaji, R; Kohara, N; Murase, N; Ikeda, A; Shibasaki, H, Iizuka, T. Movement-related cortical potentials before jaw excursions in oromandibular dystonia. *Mov. Disord.*, 2003;18:94-100.

[176] Yoshida, K; Kaji, R; Hamano, T; Kohara, N; Kimura, J; Iizuka T. Cortical distribution of Bereitschaftspotential and negative slope potential preceding mouth opening movements in human subjects. *Arch. Oral Biol.*, 1999;44:183-190.

[177] Hamano, T; Lüders, HO; Ikeda, A; Collura, TF; Comair, YG; Shibasaki, H. The cortical generators of the contingent negative variation in humans: a

study with subdural electrodes. *Electroencephalogr. Clin. Neurophysiol.*, 1997;104:257-268.
[178] Yazawa, S; Shibasaki, H; Ikeda, A; Terada, K; Nagamine, T; Honda, M. Cortical mechanism underlying externally cued gait initiation studied by contingent negative variation. *Electroencephalogr. Clin. Neurophysiol.*, 1997;105:390-399.
[179] Lai, C; Ikeda, A; Terada, K; Nagamine, T; Honda, M; Xu, X; Yoshimura, N; Howng, S; Barrett, G; Shibasaki, H. Event-related potentials associated with judgment: comparison of S1 and S2 choice conditions in a contingent negative variation (CNV) paradigm. *J. Clin. Neurophysiol.*, 1997;14:394-405.
[180] Cui, RQ; Egkher, A; Huter, D; Lang, W; Lindinger, G; Deecke, L. High resolution spatiotemporal analysis of the contingent negative variation in simple or complex motor tasks and a non-motor task. *Clin. Neurophysiol.*, 2000;111:1847-1859.
[181] Oishi, M; Mochizuki, Y. Correlation between contingent negative variation and movement-related cortical potentials in parkinsonism. *Electroencephalogr. Clin. Neurophysiol.*, 1995;95:346-349.
[182] Lamarche, M; Louvel, J; Buser, P; Rektor, I. Intracerebral recordings of slow potentials in a contingent negative variation paradigm: in exploration in epileptic patients. *Electroencephalogr. Clin. Neurophysiol.*, 1995;95:268-276.
[183] Delse, FC; Marsh, GR; Thompson, LW. CNV correlates of task difficulty and accuracy of pitch discrimination. *Psychophysiology*, 1972;9:139-154.
[184] Low, MD; McSherry, JW. Further observations of psychological factors involved in CNV genesis. *Electroencephalogr. Clin. Neurophysiol.*, 1968;25:203-207.
[185] Nakamura, M; Fukui, Y; Kadobayashi, I; Kato, N. A comparison of the CNV in young and old subjects: its relation to memory and personality. *Electroencephalogr. Clin. Neurophysiol.*, 1979;46:337-344.
[186] Glanzmann, P; Froehlich, WD. Anxiety, stress, and contingent negative variation reconsidered. *Ann. N. Y. Acad. Sci.*, 1984;425:578-584.
[187] Ikeda, A; Shibasaki, H; Kaji, R; Terada, K; Nagamine, T; Honda, M; Hamano, T; Kimura, J. Abnormal sensorimotor integration in writer's cramp: study of contingent negative variation. *Mov. Disord.*, 1996;11:683-960.
[188] Nakajima, I; Miyauchi, M; Minowa, K; Akasaka, M; Uchida, A. Contingent negative variations associated with jaw opening in humans. *Somatosensory Motor. Res.*, 1994;11:149-152.

[189] Ohsawa, K; Yamaguchi, T; Murata, N; Kanazawa, K; Uchida, A; Nakajima, I. Contingent negative variations associated with vocalization in humans. *No To Shinkei*, 1996;48:357-361.

[190] Nagai, Y; Critchley, HD; Featherstone, E; Fenwick, PB; Trimble, MR; Dolan, RJ. Brain activity relating to the contingent negative variation: an fMRI investigation. *Neuroimage*, 2004;21:1232-1241.

[191] McAdam, DW; Seale, DM. Bereitschaftspotential enhancement with increased level of motivation. *Electroencephalogr. Clin. Neurophysiol.*, 1969;27:73-75.

[192] Yoshida, K; Kaji, R; Kubori, T; Kohara, N; Iizuka, T; Kimura, J. Muscle afferent block for the treatment of oromandibular dystonia. *Mov. Disord.*, 1998;13:699-705.

[193] Yoshida, K; Kaji, R; Shibasaki, H; Iizuka, T. Factors influence the therapeutic effect of muscle afferent block for oromandibular dystonia and dyskinesia: implications for their distinct pathophysiology. *Int. J. Oral. Maxillofac. Surg.*, 2002;31:499-505.

[194] Yoshida, K; Iizuka, T. Jaw deviation dystonia evaluated by movement-related cortical potentials and treated with muscle afferent block. *J. Craniomandib. Pract.*, 2003;21:295-300.

[195] Penfield, W; Rasmussen, T. *The cerebral cortex of man: a clinical study of localization of function*. New York: Macmillan; 1952.

[196] McCarthy, G.; Allison, T; Spencer, DD. Localization of the face area of human sensorimotor cortex by intracranial recording of somatosensory evoked potentials. *J. Neurosurg*, 1993;79:874-884.

[197] Karhu, J; Hari, R; Lu, S; Paetau, R; Rif, J. Neuromagnetic responses to lingual nerve stimulation. *Electroencephalogr. Clin. Neurophysiol.*, 1991;80:459-468.

[198] Hari, R; Karhu, J; Hämäläinen, M; Knuutila, J; Salonen, O; Sams, M; Vilkman, V. Functional organization of the human first and second somatosensory cortices: a neuromagnetic study. *Eur. J. Neurosci.*, 1993;5:724-734.

[199] Nakamura, A; Yamada, T; Goto, A; Kato, T; Ito, K; Abe, Y; Kachi, T; Kakigi, R. Somatosensory homunculus as drawn by MEG. *Neuroimage*, 1998;7:377-386.

[200] Yamashita, H; Kumamoto, Y; Nakashima, T; Yamamoto, T; Inokuchi, A; Komiyama, S. Magnetic sensory cortical responses evoked by tactile stimulations of the human face, oral cavity and flap reconstructions of the tongue. *Eur. Arch. Otorhinolaryngol.*, 1999;256(Suppl 1):S42-S46.

[201] Kakigi, R; Hoshiyama, M; Shimojo, M; Naka, D; Yamasaki, H; Watanabe, S; Xiang, J; Maeda, K; Lam, K; Itomi, K; Nakamura, A. The somatosensory evoked magnetic fields. *Prog. Neurobiol.*, 2000;61:495-523.
[202] Suzuki, T; Shibukawa, Y; Kumai, T; Shintani, M. Face area representation of primary somatosensory cortex in humans identified by whole-head magnetoencephalography. *Jpn. J. Physiol.*, 2004;54:161-169.
[203] Nakahara, H; Nakasato, N; Kanno, A; Murayama, S; Hatanaka, K; Itoh, H; Yoshimoto, T. Somatosensory-evoked fields for gingival, lip, and tongue. *J. Dent. Res.*, 2004;83,:307-311.
[204] Nguyen, BT; Inui, K; Hoshiyama, M; Nakata, H; Kakigi, R. Face representation in the human secondary somatosensory cortex. *Clin. Neurophysiol.*, 2005;116:1247-1253.
[205] Lotze, M; Seggewies, G; Erb, M; Grodd, W; Birbaumer, N. The representation of articulation in the primary sensorimotor cortex. *Neuroreport*, 2000;11:2985-2989.
[206] Ettlin, DA; Zhang, H; Lutz, K; Jarmann, T; Meier, D; Gallo, LM; Jancke, L; Palla, S. Cortical activation resulting from painless vibrotactile dental stimulation measured by functional magnetic resonance imaging (fMRI). *J. Dent. Res.*, 2004;83:757-761.
[207] Miyamoto, JJ; Honda, M; Saito, DN; Okada, T; Ono, T; Ohyama, K; Sadato, N. The representation of the human oral area in the somatosensory cortex: a functional MRI study. *Cereb. Cortex*, 2006;16:669-675.
[208] Civardi, C; Naldi, P; Cantello, R. Cortico-motoneurone excitability in patients with obstructive sleep apnoea. *J. Sleep Res.*, 2004;13:159-163.
[209] Friberg, D; Gazelius, B; Hokfelt, T; Nordlander, B. Abnormal afferent nerve endings in the soft palatal mucosa of sleep apneics and habitual snorers. *Regul. Pept.*, 1997;71:29-36.
[210] Friberg, D; Ansved, T; Borg, K; Carlsson-Nordlander, B; Larsson, H; Svanborg, E. Histological indications of a progressive snorers disease in an upper airway muscle. *Am. J. Respir. Crit. Care Med.*, 1998;157:586-593.
[211] Kimoff, RJ; Sforza, E; Champagne, V; Ofiara, L; Gendron, D. Upper airway sensation in snoring and obstructive sleep apnea. *Am. J. Respir. Crit. Care Med.*, 2001;164:250-255.
[212] Guilleminault, C; Li, K; Chen, NH; Poyares, D. Two-point palatal discrimination in patients with upper airway resistance syndrome, obstructive sleep apnea syndrome, and normal control subjects. *Chest*, 2002;122:866-870.

[213] Hashimoto, I. From input to output in the somatosensory system for natural air-puff stimulation of the skin. *Electroencephalogr. Clin. Neurophysiol.*, 1999; 49(Suppl):269-283.

[214] Ahonen, AI; Hämäläinen, MS; Kajola, MJ; Knuutila, JET; Laine, PP; Lounasmaa, OV; Simola, J; Tesche, C; Vilkman, V. 122-channel SQUID instrument for investigating the magnetic signals from the human brain. *Physica Scripta*, 1993;T49,198-205.

[215] Nagamine, T; Kajola, M; Salmelin, R; Shibasaki, H; Hari, R. Movement-related slow cortical magnetic fields and changes of spontaneous MEG- and EEG-brain rhythms. *Electroenceph. Clin. Neurophysiol.*, 1996;99:274-286.

[216] Hämäläinen, M; Hari, R; Ilmoniemi, RJ; Knuutila, J; Lounasmaa, OV. Magnetoencephalography-theory, instrumentation, and applications to noninvasive studies of the working human brain. *Rev. Mod. Phys.*, 1993;65:413-498.

[217] Maloney, SR; Bell, WL; Shoaf, SC; Blair, D; Bastings, EP; Good, DC; Quinlivan, L. Measurement of lingual and palatine somatosensory evoked potentials. *Clin. Neurophysiol.*, 2000;111:291-296.

[218] McCarthy, G; Allison, T. Trigeminal evoked potentials in somatosensory cortex of the Macaca mulatta. *J. Neurosurg.*, 1995;82:1015-1020.

[219] Maeda, K; Kakigi, R; Hoshiyama, M; Koyama, S. Topography of the secondary somatosensory cortex in humans: a magnetoencephalographic study. *Neuroreport*, 1999;10:301-306.

[220] Loose, R; Schnitzler, A; Sarkar, S; Schmitz, F; Volkmann, J; Frieling, T; Freund, HJ; Witte, OW; Enck, P. Cortical activation during oesophageal stimulation: a neuromagnetic study. *Neurogastroenterol. Mot.*, 1999;11:163-171.

[221] Schnitzler, A; Volkmann, J; Enck, P; Frieling, T; Witte, OW; Freund, HJ. Different cortical organization of visceral and somatic sensation in humans. *Eur. J. Neurosci.*, 1999;11:305-315.

[222] Hari, R; Forss, N. Magnetoencephalography in the study of human somatosensory cortical processing. *Phil. Trans. R. Soc. Lond.*, 1999; 354: 1145-1154.

[223] Birn, RM; Bandettini, PA; Cox, RW; Shaker, R. Event-related fMRI of tasks involving brief motion. *Hum. Brain Mapp.*, 1999;7:106-114.

[224] Chance, B; Zhuang, Z; UnAh, C; Alter, C; Lipton, L. Cognition-activated low-frequency modulation of light absorption in human brain. *Proc. Natl. Acad. Sci. USA*, 1993;90:3770-3774.

[225] Strangman, G; Culver, JP; Thompson, JH; Boas, DA. A quantitative comparison of simultaneous BOLD fMRI and NIRS recordings during functional brain activation. *Neuroimage*, 2002;17:719-731.
[226] Miyamoto, I; Yoshida, K; Tsuboi, Y; Iizuka, T. Rehabilitation with dental prosthesis can increase cerebral regional blood flow. *Clin. Oral Impl. Res.*, 2005;16:723-727.
[227] Frostig, RD; Lieke, EE; Ts'o, DY; Grinvald, A. Cortical functional architecture and local coupling between neuronal activity and the microcirculation revealed by in vivo high-resolution optical imaging of intrinsic signals. *Proc. Natl. Acad. Sci. USA.*, 1990;87:6082-6086.
[228] Villringer, A; Chance, B. Non-invasive optical spectroscopy and imaging of human brain function. *Trends Neurosci.*, 1997,20:435-442.
[229] Penfield, W; Boldrey, E. Somatic motor and sensory representation in the cerebral cortex of man as studied by electrical stimulation. *Brain*, 1937;60:389-443.
[230] Nakamura, Y; Katakura, N. Generation of masticatory rhythm in the brainstem. *Neurosci. Res.*, 1995;23:1-19.
[231] Catania, KC; Remple, MS. Somatosensory cortex dominated by the representation of teeth in the naked mole-rat brain. *Proc. Natl. Acad. Sci. USA.*, 2002;99:5692-5697.
[232] Godde, B; Berkefeld, T; David-Jurgens, M; Dinse, HR. Age-related changes in primary somatosensory cortex of rats: evidence for parallel degenerative and plastic-adaptive processes. *Neurosci. Biobehav. Rev.*, 2002;26:743-752.
[233] Terasawa, H; Hirai, T; Ninomiya, T; Ikeda, Y; Ishijima, T; Yajima, T; Hamaue, N; Nagase, Y; Kang, Y; Minami, M. Influence of tooth-loss and concomitant masticatory alterations on cholinergic neurons in rats: immunohistochemical and biochemical studies. *Neurosci. Res.*, 2002;43:373-379.
[234] Ikeda, M; Brown, J; Holland, AJ; Fukuhara, R; Hodges, JR. Changes in appetite, food preference, and eating habits in frontotemporal dementia and Alzheimer's disease. *J. Neurol. Neurosurg. Psychiatry*, 2002;73:371-376.
[235] Eker, C; Hagstadius, S; Linden, A; Schalen, W; Nordstrom, CH. Neuropsychological assessments in relation to CBF after severe head injuries. *Act Neurol. Scand.*, 2001;104:142-147.
[236] Décary, A; Rouleau, I; Montplaisir, J. Cognitive deficits associated with sleep apnea syndrome: a proposed neurophychological test battery. *Sleep*, 2000;23:369-381.

[237] Fulda, S; Schulz, H. Cognitive dysfunction in sleep disorders. *Sleep Med. Rev.*, 2001;5:423-445.
[238] Jones, K; Harrison, Y. Frontal lobe function, sleep loss and fragmented sleep. *Sleep Med. Rev.*, 2001;5:463-475.
[239] Suto, T; Fukuda, M; Ito, M; Uehara, T; Mikuni, M. Multichannel near-infrared spectroscopy in depression and schizophrenia: cognitive brain activation study. *Biol. Psychiatry*, 2004;55:501-511.

INDEX

A

ablations, 129
abnormalities, ix, 82, 92, 111, 115, 117
absorption, 61, 138
accidents, 2, 115
accuracy, 134
activation, 71, 80, 102, 103, 105, 107, 129, 136, 138, 140
acute, 31, 124
adaptation, 53
adipocytes, 58
adipose tissue, 59
adjustment, 15, 36, 48, 49
adult, 2, 127
adulthood, 112
adults, 23, 53, 54, 115, 122, 126
afferent nerve, 136
Ag, 66
age, 7, 22, 26, 34, 38, 43, 56, 59, 82, 90, 95
aggregates, 57
agonist, 71
air, 8, 11, 13, 58, 63, 95, 96, 97, 99, 101, 102, 103, 129, 137
airways, 17, 37, 122
alcohol, 60
algorithm, 75
alpha, 21, 128
alpha activity, 21
alternative, 11, 33

amplitude, 63, 69, 70, 72, 75, 77, 78, 79, 80, 82, 84, 87, 88, 90, 91, 92, 99
analysis of variance, 75, 84
anatomy, 3, 37, 38, 113, 116
angina, 2, 115
ANOVA, 31, 45, 75, 77, 84, 87
ANS, 18
antagonist, 71
anthropology, 3
antihypertensive drugs, 31
anxiety, 111
Anxiety, 134
apnea, iv, ix, x, 1, 7, 9, 10, 19, 21, 23, 26, 31, 38, 39, 44, 45, 46, 47, 48, 50, 63, 68, 69, 70, 71, 72, 115, 116, 124, 125, 126, 129
appetite, 139
arousal, 21, 24, 27, 31, 34, 35, 36, 81
arrhythmias, 9
ARS, 34
arterial hypertension, 2, 25, 31
arteriosclerosis, 57, 59
artery, 2, 115
arthralgia, 21
articulation, 136
Asia, 59
asphyxia, 31
assessment, 94, 118, 130
atherogenesis, 54, 55
atherosclerosis, 60
attachment, 10, 11
averaging, 74, 84, 97, 108, 130

B

bacteremia, 59
bacteria, 54, 55, 59
basal ganglia, 82, 91
battery, 139
behavior, 109, 111
beneficial effect, 38, 48
benefits, 10
bias, 124
biofilms, 55
bleeding, 55
blood, 1, 26, 27, 28, 29, 30, 31, 32, 33, 55, 57, 62, 63, 90, 93, 104, 105, 106, 109, 121, 122, 123, 124, 138
blood pressure, 26, 27, 28, 29, 30, 31, 32, 33, 62, 121, 122, 123, 124
blood pressure reduction, 31, 33
blood stream, 55
BMI, 26
body mass index, 22, 26, 34, 38, 45, 95
body weight, 27, 112
BOLD, 138
bolus, 74
bone graft, 53
bone loss, 55
brain, x, 63, 65, 94, 98, 102, 104, 105, 106, 109, 111, 130, 132, 137, 138, 139, 140
brain activity, x, 104, 105
brainstem, 139
breathing, x, 3, 11, 14, 15, 32, 34, 51, 52, 61, 63, 71, 72, 113, 115, 116, 119, 122, 126
bruxism, 56, 58, 61
buccal mucosa, 10

C

caliber, 12, 20, 33
calorie, 7
cancer, 60
candidates, 32
carbon, 1
carbon dioxide, 1
cardiovascular disease, 60, 128
cardiovascular morbidity, 31
cast, 14, 95
catecholamines, 122
Caucasian, 4
Caucasians, 3, 4
causation, 126
cavities, 3
central nervous system, 65, 94
central sleep apnea, 68, 69
cerebral blood flow, 93, 104, 110
cerebral blood volume, 105
cerebral cortex, ix, 65, 135, 139
channels, 105, 108, 109
chewing, ix, 4, 5, 7, 65, 74, 80, 105, 106, 113
childhood, 7, 113
children, ix, 53, 127
chloride, 74
cholinergic, 139
cholinergic neurons, 139
chronic obstructive pulmonary disease, 60
chronic renal failure, 60
cingulated, 91
circadian, 122
cirrhosis, 60
clinical neurophysiology, 131
closure, ix, 1
CNV, 81, 84, 86, 87, 88, 89, 90, 91, 92, 93, 132, 133, 134
Cochrane, 122
coffee, 58
cognition, 82, 107
cognitive dysfunction, 1, 110
cognitive process, ix, 65, 81
cohort, 126
complexity, 80, 90, 130
compliance, 8, 32, 34, 36, 49, 64
complications, 2, 9, 11, 37, 49, 63
components, 73, 79, 81, 101
computed tomography, 20
concentration, 105, 106, 108, 109, 110, 111
conduction, 91
confidence, 98
configuration, 50
Congress, 116
construction, 10
contamination, 78, 79, 89

continuous positive airway pressure, 7, 117, 118, 122, 123
control, ix, 20, 25, 33, 39, 62, 65, 73, 80, 81, 92, 93, 98, 99, 100, 101, 111, 137
controlled trials, 20, 25, 26, 32
conversion, 97
coronary artery disease, 2, 115
coronary heart disease, 31, 57, 59, 124
correlation, 48, 59, 110
correlations, 29
cortex, 90, 94, 102, 105, 108, 109, 110, 129, 131, 135, 136, 137, 139
cortical neurons, 105
cortical processing, 138
coupling, 138
CPAP, 7, 9, 15, 16, 17, 22, 25, 26, 32, 33, 34, 37, 47, 49, 56, 62, 63, 117, 122
craniofacial, ix, 2, 4, 5, 7, 53, 60, 112, 113, 127
cranium, 3, 106
C-reactive protein, 128
cross-sectional, 20
CRP, 59
cyst, 50
cytokines, 54, 55, 58

D

DBP, 30
de novo, 53
death, 2, 59, 124, 126
decay, 110
decision making, 82, 89, 132
defects, 58
deficiency, 53
deficits, 139
definition, 25
deformities, 53, 127
delivery, 96
dementia, 110, 139
dentist, 10, 36, 49, 61
dentistry, 62, 119, 128
dentists, 61, 62
dentures, 16
deoxyhemoglobin, 105

depression, 1, 111, 140
derivatives, 97
dermoid cyst, 50
destruction, 58
detection, 106
deviation, 135
diabetes, 56, 57, 58, 60, 62, 128
diabetes mellitus, 56, 57, 58, 60, 62
diastolic blood pressure, 26, 32, 33
diastolic pressure, 33
diet, 56
digestion, 65
dilation, 125
diodes, 83
dipole, 98, 100, 101
dipole moment, 98, 100, 101
discomfort, 8, 10, 11, 14, 15, 36, 48, 61, 63
discrimination, 134, 137
disease progression, 61
diseases, 54, 55, 56, 57, 58, 60, 62, 93
disorder, ix, 2, 36, 72, 94, 122, 126
displacement, 33, 35, 47, 71
distraction, ix, 53, 127, 128
distress, 127
distribution, 30, 63, 77, 78, 79, 81, 88, 89, 91, 100, 133
dominance, 91
dorsolateral prefrontal cortex, 82
drinking, 58
drying, 58
duration, 21, 23, 27, 29, 31, 32, 39, 40, 42, 83, 96
dyskinesia, 93, 135
dystonia, 82, 92, 132, 133, 135

E

ears, 83
eating, 7, 60, 109, 139
eating behavior, 109
EEG, 73, 74, 75, 83, 84, 105, 131, 137
elasticity, 70
electrodes, 66, 67, 71, 74, 77, 79, 83, 89, 91, 133
electroencephalography, 107, 108

electromyographic study, 130
electromyography, 129
EMG, 66, 67, 69, 70, 71, 72, 73, 74, 75, 76, 80, 83, 85, 89, 91, 105, 131
emission, 93, 104
endocarditis, 59
endocardium, 59
endothelium, 59
endotoxins, 54, 55
England, 21
environmental factors, 4
EOG, 83, 85
epiglottis, 48
epilepsy, 90
epithelium, 94
equivalent current dipole, 98, 100
ERPs, 131
Europeans, 2
event-related potential, 81
evoked potential, 94, 135, 137
excitability, 136
executive functions, 111
exercise, 60
expertise, 35, 36
extensor, 83, 85
extensor digitorum, 83, 85
extraction, 59
eye movement, 24, 41, 43, 46, 74, 84

frontotemporal dementia, 139
functional architecture, 106, 138
functional aspects, ix, 37
functional magnetic resonance imaging, 93, 104, 136
functional MRI, 94, 136

G

gait, 133
ganglia, 82, 91
gauge, 66, 67
gel, 83
general anesthesia, 19
General Electric, 97
generation, 82, 89, 90, 91, 132
generators, 90, 91, 133
genioplasty, 52
Germany, 14, 95
gingival, 55, 58, 61, 136
glucose metabolism, 58
Gram-negative, 55
gravity, 47
groups, 10, 27, 30, 39, 42, 45, 46
growth, ix, 4, 7, 112, 113
guidance, 10
guidelines, 7, 15, 35
gyrus, 82, 91, 102

F

fabrication, 36
facial muscles, 89
failure, 23, 27, 38
fat, 2, 17, 37, 57
fatigue, 34
feet, 82
fibers, 66, 94, 105, 106
films, 20
Finland, 97
flow, 90, 93, 104, 110, 138
fMRI, 104, 105, 134, 136, 138
food, 4, 7, 139
frontal cortex, 82, 89, 90
frontal lobe, 63, 89, 112

H

habituation, 21, 27, 34, 38, 48, 90
handedness, 130
hands, 55, 82
harm, 53
harmony, 53
head injuries, 139
healing, 53
health, 49, 60
hearing, 83
heart, 26, 27, 31, 57, 59, 60, 124
heart disease, 31, 57, 59, 60
heart rate, 26, 27
height, 3
hemisphere, 79, 80, 81, 91

hemodynamics, 108, 110
hemoglobin, 105, 128
hepatocytes, 59
heredity, 4
high blood pressure, 32, 57
high-speed, 101
Holland, 139
Honda, 132, 133, 134, 136
hospital, 26, 61
human, 73, 94, 121, 122, 129, 130, 131, 132, 133, 135, 136, 137, 138
human brain, 132, 137, 138
human subjects, 121, 133
humans, 65, 89, 102, 109, 129, 130, 132, 133, 134, 136, 138
hygiene, 61, 128
hyoid, 2, 17, 18, 19, 20, 37, 50, 51, 66, 120
hyperglycemia, 58
hyperlipemia, 62
hyperlipidemia, 57, 60
hypersomnia, 129
hypertension, 30, 31, 32, 57, 60, 115, 122, 124
Hypertension, 30, 34, 56, 123
hypertensive, 26, 31, 32
hypertrophy, 2, 17, 37
hypocapnia, 72
hypopnea, 21, 22, 28, 30, 40, 42, 123
hypothesis, 94, 103, 126
hypotonia, 71
hypoventilation, 72
hypoxemia, 111
hypoxia, 110

I

id, 30, 72
idiopathic, 133
images, 65, 100, 104, 110
imaging, 20, 91, 93, 104, 105, 120, 136, 138
imaging modalities, 20
imaging techniques, 93
immunohistochemical, 139
impacted teeth, 5
impairments, 111
imperative stimulus, 81, 92

in vivo, 138
inclusion, 21, 35
indication, 15, 120, 127
indices, 39
individual differences, 48
induction, 53
infancy, 112
infection, 9, 54, 55
inflammation, 54, 55, 58, 59, 61
inflammatory, 54, 55
information processing speed, 110
infrared, 105
infrared spectroscopy, x, 63, 105, 140
inhibition, 72
initiation, 59, 133
injection, 66, 67, 104
injury, 110
insertion, 20, 22, 24, 25, 26, 27, 34, 35, 38, 39, 46, 71
insight, 101
inspections, 74
inspiration, 71
instability, 17, 37
insulin, 58, 128
insulin resistance, 59, 128
integration, 81, 92, 134
interactions, 84, 87
interleukin-6, 58, 59, 128
interval, 26, 81, 83, 96
intervention, 33, 51
intracranial, 94, 102, 103, 135
intramuscular, ix, 65
intravenous, 104
intrinsic, 138
invasive, 129, 138
ipsilateral, 79, 80, 81, 91, 103

J

JAMA, 119, 128
Japan, 2, 11, 14, 26, 58, 60, 66, 74, 96, 105, 107
Japanese, 2, 3, 4, 5, 17, 58, 60, 128
jaw, ix, 9, 10, 53, 62, 63, 65, 73, 80, 82, 83, 84, 87, 90, 91, 104, 129, 133, 134

joint pain, 36
joints, 80
judgment, 89, 133

L

laser, 50, 106
latency, 25, 34, 81, 98, 99, 100, 101, 102, 103, 125
laterality, 103
law, 106
learning, 109
left hemisphere, 77, 91
leptin, 58
lesions, 59
lifestyle, 56, 57, 58, 60, 61, 62
life-threatening, 9
light emitting diode, 83
limitations, 109
linear, 31
lingual, 14, 92, 135, 137
lipopolysaccharides, 55
liver, 60
liver disease, 60
localization, 93, 105, 135
long distance, 53
longitudinal study, 49
lumen, 94

M

macroglossia, 17, 50, 51
macrophages, 58
magnetic, 63, 91, 94, 96, 97, 98, 100, 129, 137
magnetic field, 63, 94, 96, 97, 98, 129, 135, 137
magnetic resonance, 93, 100, 104, 136
magnetic resonance imaging, 93, 104, 136
magnetoencephalography, x, 104, 136
maintenance, 25
malocclusion, 7
management, 8, 10, 112, 126
mandible, 3, 6, 7, 10, 11, 13, 16, 17, 19, 20, 33, 35, 36, 37, 46, 47, 52, 54, 63, 66, 70, 71, 72, 119

mandibular, 2, 3, 5, 6, 8, 10, 11, 12, 14, 17, 19, 20, 33, 36, 37, 47, 50, 51, 53, 65, 73, 77, 79, 80, 81, 82, 83, 90, 116, 117, 118, 119, 120, 121, 127, 129
mapping, 94
mask, 8, 97
masseter, 20, 46, 66, 67, 68, 69, 70, 71, 74, 83, 85, 89, 129
mastication, 109, 129, 130
masticatory, 5, 16, 33, 35, 36, 37, 63, 65, 66, 71, 72, 75, 76, 79, 87, 89, 92, 105, 108, 109, 121, 124, 139
maxilla, 6, 52
maxillary, 5, 10, 11, 12, 14, 51, 53, 66, 95
maxillary sinus, 53
MBP, 30
mean arterial blood pressure, 26, 31
mean arterial pressure, 27, 29, 31, 32, 33
measurement, 25, 26, 32, 63, 96, 98, 105, 106, 107, 117
measures, 84
median, 49
mediators, 54, 55
medical care, 55
medication, 26, 32
medicine, 62, 118, 119, 122, 126, 128
MEG, 93, 97, 104, 105, 135, 137
memory, 1, 82, 109, 111, 134
memory capacity, 110
memory loss, 2
men, 22, 26, 34, 38, 45, 66, 82, 95, 115, 116, 128
mental health, 60
mental states, 82
mentally impaired, 10, 119
meta-analysis, 124
metabolic, 57, 60, 128
metabolic syndrome, 57, 60, 128
metabolism, 58
mice, 128
microcirculation, 138
microorganisms, 55
Microsoft, 75
middle-aged, 2, 115, 128
modalities, ix, 20

modality, 132
models, 12
modulation, 138
mole, 139
monkeys, 65, 102
monocytes, 58
morbidity, 9, 31, 56
morning, 14, 21, 31, 34, 36, 124
morphology, 2, 3, 4, 5, 7, 60, 112, 113
mortality, 31, 128
motion, 21, 65, 72, 104, 138
motivation, 134
motor area, 65, 79, 90, 91
motor control, 82
motor task, 92, 133
mouth, 1, 3, 14, 21, 33, 35, 36, 47, 58, 61, 63, 66, 71, 74, 75, 76, 77, 78, 79, 80, 83, 85, 86, 87, 88, 89, 90, 91, 95, 96, 97, 98, 100, 106, 108, 131, 133
movement, ix, 9, 10, 11, 21, 36, 62, 63, 65, 66, 73, 74, 75, 76, 77, 78, 79, 80, 82, 83, 84, 85, 86, 87, 88, 89, 90, 91, 92, 105, 130, 131, 132, 133, 134, 135
MRI, 12, 93, 94, 97, 98, 104, 136
mucosa, 10, 58, 94, 96, 136
mucous membranes, 49
muscle, 1, 14, 15, 16, 19, 20, 38, 46, 47, 48, 63, 66, 67, 69, 70, 71, 72, 74, 78, 80, 83, 84, 89, 91, 92, 105, 121, 124, 130, 135, 137
muscle contraction, 72, 92
muscles, ix, 5, 17, 20, 33, 35, 36, 37, 38, 46, 65, 66, 67, 68, 69, 70, 71, 72, 75, 76, 77, 79, 80, 83, 87, 89, 94, 105, 129
myocardial infarction, 31, 54, 55, 124

N

nares, 117
nasopharynx, 11, 25
natural, 101, 137
near-infrared spectroscopy, x, 63, 105, 140
neck, 92
necrosis, 58, 128
negativity, 73, 75, 76, 80, 84, 85, 88, 91, 132
nephritis, 60
nerve, 94, 102, 135
neurological disorder, 94
neurons, 129, 139
New York, 115, 125, 135
NIH, 121
NIRS, 107, 111, 112, 138
nitrogen, 96
noise, 97, 101
non-invasive, 63, 105
normal, ix, 3, 7, 46, 53, 71, 93, 95, 101, 112, 113, 137
novelty, 80
nucleus, 82

O

obese, 2, 17, 47, 48, 50, 57, 58, 60, 116
obesity, 2, 7, 48, 56, 57, 58, 59, 60, 61, 113, 128
observations, 134
obstruction, ix, 1, 2, 3, 4, 8, 9, 17, 35, 37, 38, 47, 48, 50, 53, 63, 71, 126, 127
obstructive sleep apnea, ix, 7, 33, 66, 68, 115, 116, 117, 118, 119, 120, 121, 122, 123, 124, 125, 126, 127, 137
occipital regions, 90
occlusion, 3, 36, 49, 125
oil, 97
optical, 105, 106, 138
optical imaging, 138
optical properties, 105
oral, ix, 7, 10, 11, 12, 15, 16, 17, 19, 20, 21, 23, 25, 26, 27, 31, 32, 33, 34, 36, 38, 39, 44, 45, 47, 49, 50, 54, 55, 58, 59, 61, 62, 63, 65, 66, 70, 94, 102, 105, 112, 118, 119, 120, 121, 123, 124, 125, 130, 135, 136
oral cavity, 49, 50, 56, 61, 102, 135
oral hygiene, 61
oral surgeon, 50
organ, 109
orientation, 98, 100
oropharyngeal region, 2
oropharynx, 2, 17, 20, 37, 62, 71
orthopaedic, 120
OSA, 120

osteoporosis, 60
osteotomy, 50, 51, 52
overeating, 7, 113
oxygen, 21, 23, 27, 28, 30, 35, 39, 40, 42, 104, 105, 116
oxygen saturation, 21, 23, 27, 28, 30, 35, 39, 40, 42, 105
oxygenation, 46
oxyhemoglobin, 105, 111, 112

P

pain, 9, 16, 21, 36
palate, 1, 3, 10, 12, 17, 19, 20, 37, 47, 48, 49, 53, 63, 94, 95, 96, 97, 98, 99, 100, 101, 102, 103, 104, 129
pancreatic, 122
parkinsonism, 132, 134
passive, 35, 47, 128
pathogenesis, 31, 37, 101
pathogens, 54, 55
pathophysiology, 82, 92, 135
pathways, 95
pediatric, 8
perception, 35, 62, 94, 95, 101, 103
periodicity, 70, 72
periodontal, 55, 56, 57, 58, 59, 61, 62
periodontal disease, 55, 56, 57, 58, 59, 61, 62
periodontitis, 54, 55, 128
periodontium, 55
personal relations, 111
personality, 134
PET, 104
pharyngeal airway, 20
pharynx, 49, 102
Philadelphia, 118, 119, 122, 126
phonation, 107, 131
physical activity, 60
physiological, 82, 92, 95, 101
physiology, 37, 113
pitch, 134
placebo, 20, 32, 123
planar, 97
plastic, 106, 139
platysma, 71

play, 47, 82
PMA, 116
polypeptide, 122
polysomnography, 2, 25, 34, 35, 48
polyurethane, 66, 67
polyvinylchloride, 96
poor, 38, 48, 64, 93, 105
population, 2, 17, 32, 54, 60, 110, 124
positive correlation, 90
positron, 93, 104
positron emission tomography, 93, 104
postoperative, 9, 52
posture, 38, 44, 47, 48, 106, 125
power, 63
prediction, 48
predictors, 120
preference, 74, 130, 139
prefrontal cortex, 82, 132
pressure, 1, 7, 11, 16, 19, 26, 27, 28, 29, 30, 31, 32, 33, 34, 35, 47, 57, 62, 63, 94, 117, 118, 121, 122, 123, 124
prevention, 7, 60, 113
probe, 106
production, 59, 131
prognosis, 116
pronunciation, 63
prosthesis, 110, 138
protection, 31
protein, 59
protocol, 50, 51
psychiatric disorders, 111
psychiatrists, 111
public health, 25
pulse, 98
purification, 61

Q

questionnaire, 35

R

range, 9, 22, 27, 32, 45, 46, 49, 95, 98
rapid eye movement sleep, 23, 24, 35, 38, 39
rats, 139

reaction time, 90
reasoning, 110
receptors, 20, 33
reconstruction, 51
redundancy, 49
reflection, 106
regression, 124
regular, 36, 48
relapse, 38
relationship, 11, 46, 57, 60, 109
relaxation, 47, 72
relevance, 62
renal, 60
resin, 14, 96
resistance, 15, 33, 34, 36, 47, 58, 59, 71, 119, 125, 128, 137
resolution, 93, 104, 105, 112, 133, 138
respiration, 58, 65, 71
respiratory, ix, 2, 11, 17, 27, 29, 34, 35, 37, 46, 47, 52, 62, 63, 72, 94, 95, 101, 110, 117, 121, 125, 127, 131
retention, 15
returns, 1
rhythm, 137, 139
right hemisphere, 77, 98, 100
risk, 2, 25, 31, 47, 49, 54, 55, 57, 58, 60, 122
risk factors, 58
Rouleau, 139

S

SAC, 21
safety, 34
saliva, 7, 61
sampling, 74, 84, 97
SAS, 1, 2, 4, 7, 8, 9, 10, 15, 16, 17, 18, 20, 25, 26, 31, 32, 38, 49, 50, 51, 52, 54, 55, 56, 57, 58, 60, 61, 62, 63, 66, 70, 71, 93, 94, 105, 110, 111, 112, 113, 117
satisfaction, 8
saturation, 21, 23, 27, 28, 30, 35, 39, 40, 42, 105
SBP, 30
scalp, 74, 82, 83, 84, 91, 97, 105, 130, 131
scalp topography, 130

schizophrenia, 140
scores, 34
secrete, 58
secretion, 7
SEFs, 94, 103
sensation, 8, 64, 95, 137, 138
sensorimotor cortex, 135, 136
separation, 14, 36, 49, 53
septum, 3
sequelae, 2
serum, 59
severity, 31, 38, 48, 126
sex, 30
side effects, 8, 14, 36
sign, 131
signals, 66, 83, 97, 106, 137, 138
SII, 100, 101, 102, 103
silver, 74
similarity, 92
sinus, 3
sites, 17, 37, 84, 97, 103
skin, 83, 137
sleep apnea, ix, 3, 7, 9, 10, 17, 37, 39, 56, 57, 62, 63, 66, 68, 72, 94, 113, 115, 116, 117, 118, 119, 121, 122, 123, 124, 125, 126, 127, 129, 139
sleep stage, 125
sleep-disordered breathing, 11, 15, 32, 34, 51, 52, 113, 115, 118, 119, 122, 126
slow-wave, 23
smoking, 60
snoring, ix, 1, 7, 8, 9, 10, 11, 13, 15, 20, 25, 34, 46, 50, 56, 58, 61, 113, 115, 116, 117, 118, 119, 121, 126, 137
soft palate, 1, 10, 12, 17, 19, 20, 37, 47, 48, 49, 63, 94, 95, 96, 97, 98, 99, 100, 101, 102, 103, 104, 129
somatosensory, 63, 94, 96, 100, 102, 103, 109, 135, 136, 137, 138, 139
somatosensory evoked magnetic fields, 94, 136
somnolence, 1
sounds, 17, 21, 36
spatial, 93, 104
spatiotemporal, 108, 110, 133

specialization, 131
spectroscopy, 138
speech, 65, 78, 130, 131
speed, 101
spine, 18, 19
splint, 16, 121
SQUID, 137
stability, 15
stabilize, 71
stages, 21
standard deviation, 45, 77, 78
standard error, 44, 45, 87, 88
stenosis, 9
stimulus, 72, 81, 92, 96, 99, 132
strength, 98, 101, 103
stress, 53, 58, 82, 134
stroke, 31, 54, 55, 60, 124
subjective, 1, 25
success rate, 9, 21, 38, 47, 52
sudden infant death syndrome, 47, 126
sugar, 58
surface area, 55
surgery, ix, 7, 15, 17, 37, 47, 50, 51, 52, 53, 127, 128
Surgery, 49, 50, 51
surgical, ix, 7, 9, 34, 50, 52, 53, 59, 112, 119, 124, 126, 127
surgical intervention, 51
swallowing, 65
Sylvian sulcus, 102
sympathetic, 31, 124
symptoms, 2, 8, 16, 36, 48, 49, 55, 95, 111, 121
syndrome, iv, ix, 3, 7, 9, 15, 34, 51, 52, 57, 58, 60, 92, 115, 116, 117, 118, 119, 120, 121, 122, 123, 125, 126, 127, 129, 137, 139
systolic blood pressure, 26, 33

T

tactile stimuli, 95, 101
task difficulty, 134
task performance, 107
teeth, 5, 6, 16, 21, 54, 55, 56, 58, 109, 139

temporal, 80, 90, 91, 93, 99, 104, 106, 107, 108, 109, 110
tension, 3
thalamus, 82, 91
therapy, 7, 9, 11, 15, 17, 23, 25, 26, 27, 31, 32, 33, 34, 38, 47, 48, 61, 63, 112, 113, 116, 119, 120, 121, 122, 123, 124, 125
thoracic, 21
three-dimensional, 73, 83
thromboembolic, 54, 55
time resolution, 105, 112
time series, 108
timing, 31, 124
tin, 83
tissue, 2, 17, 37, 38, 50, 53, 58, 59, 105, 106
titration, 47
TNF, 58, 128
TNF-alpha, 128
Tokyo, 66, 105, 107, 116, 119, 128
Tongue, 9, 50, 85, 87, 88, 89
tonic, 80
tonsils, 50
topographic, 77
torus, 50
tracheostomy, 7, 117
training, 116
travel, 16, 49
Treacher Collins syndrome, 51
Treponema denticola, 55
trial, 33, 121, 123
trigeminal, 103
tumor, 58, 128
turbinates, 3
two-way, 84, 87
type 2 diabetes, 58, 60, 128

U

upper airways, 2
uvula, 19, 48, 50

V

values, 26, 39, 41, 43, 45, 84, 90, 106, 108
variability, 94

variables, ix, 11, 22, 23, 24, 27, 28, 29, 30, 31, 34, 39, 40, 42
variance, 75, 84
variation, ix, 62, 65, 81, 90, 109, 124, 129, 131, 132, 133, 134
vascular disease, 128
velocity, 81, 92, 101
ventilation, 1, 72
vibration, 94
vocalizations, 78, 130

W

water, 14, 104
wear, 35, 120
weight loss, 7, 47, 116
windows, 109
women, 22, 26, 34, 38, 45, 66, 82, 95, 119

Y

young adults, 23